I'LL TELL YOU LATER

I'LL TELL YOU LATER

Deaf Survivors of Dinner Table Syndrome

Raymond Luczak,
Editor

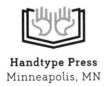

Handtype Press
Minneapolis, MN

Acknowledgments

The following reprints in this anthology are as follows:

Cristina Hartmann's "Carnaval, Update" appeared in *Peatsmoke Journal* (Spring 2021 Issue).

Raymond Luczak's "Here Lies the Body of a Deaf Boy" appeared in *Yooper Poetry: On Experiencing Michigan's Upper Peninsula* (Raymond Luczak, ed.; Modern History Press, 2024).

Kris Ringman's "Last Rites Are Never What You Expect" appeared in *Sail Skin: Poems* (Handtype Press, 2022).

John David Walker's "That Question Again" was revised from a post on his Facebook page.

Garrett Zuercher's *The Deaf Table: a short play* was originally written for Deaf Austin Theater's 2024 Short Play Festival.

Jer Loudenback's poem "Family Language" and André Pellerin's "Not Important" were translated from ASL into English by Raymond Luczak.

The editor wishes to thank Andrew J. Oehrlein Bjarnvold, Joseph L. Cumer, Arthur Durkee, Adam Kauwenberg-Marsnik, Eric Thomas Norris, André Pellerin (*in memoriam*), Tom Steele, and Les K. Wright for their assistance in ways both small and significant with this project. The memory of David Cummer (1956-2022) continues to be a blessing.

Copyright

in memoriam

André Pellerin
(1958-2024)

CONTENTS

"The most terrible loneliness is not the kind that comes from being alone, but the kind that comes from being misunderstood. It is the loneliness of standing in a crowded room, surrounded by people who do not see you, who do not hear you, who do not know the true essence of who you are. And in that loneliness, you feel as though you are fading, disappearing into the background, until you are nothing more than a ghost, a shadow of your former self."

—Attribution unknown

These Four Words

I'll ...

Whenever I sit at a table filled with hearing people who don't understand how much effort it takes to lipread and follow the staccato changes in their banter, I'm already lost at sea. I become a tugboat with no anchor to my name. The winds of banter buffer me each time I dine with them. The food on my plate and I conduct a far more meaningful conversation. It's even more painful when these very people are your own family, the ones who should know better about your own communication access needs. They should know from having seen up close the efforts you've had to make at school.

I count myself among the thousands and thousands of Deaf* people who can no longer find the umbilical cord to connect to their hearing families. We Deaf people have rarely felt respected in the houses where we grew up; in fact, we have been ignored. We are too much work. No one checks in with us to ask whether we're able to follow the conversation. They're too busy having a great time with each other. We often wonder if they've ever noticed how little we say, how rarely we laugh mainly because we can't understand them. My, my, we're just joyless siblings, aren't we?

The fact is, lipreading is hard work. Make that a *lot* of work. Hearing people aren't willing to slow down and ask whether we want to add something to the conversation.

The only hearing family story we recall more than any other is not about our siblings and relatives, but of the way we were left out of their joyful sharing between generations. We grow up with a very different family history from theirs. Because we do not know our family stories, we do not feel such a strong bond with them. Our need to feel loved *and* included at these gatherings does not matter. Our deafness have made us a duty, a chore, a slog.

---

* Throughout this anthology, the words "Deaf" (capital-D) and "deaf" (lowercase) may seem interchangeable. They are not. "Deaf" refers to those who use Sign as a primary means to communicate and do not see their own hearing loss as a pathological condition; "deaf" refers to those who do not use Sign to communicate and may view their own hearing loss as a medical issue. Either way, *both* groups have experienced Dinner Table Syndrome (DTS).

With each family meal, and with each time we do not feel included, and therefore we do not matter (*Oh, come on, you know that's not true, you're still one of us!*), the gossamer thread between us and our hearing families grow thinner until it quietly—or sometimes quite dramatically—snaps. We learn not to feel so guilty about avoiding family gatherings and reunions.

If we seem angry, it is because we know we are worthy of *full* respect as human beings. We know deep down that we deserve to be treated as equals to them. We are not family dogs.

Never mind the fact that many of us have had to spend years in speech therapy. Successful lipreading rests largely on whether we've immediately decoded the context of the conversation, praying that the speaker won't suddenly change the topic halfway. We are lost again. The more the topic changes, the more tossed about at sea we feel. At the family table, we learn to become ghosts. Our apparent insignificance at their meals continues to haunt us long after we've left home. Sometimes we ask ourselves why we even bother to return and pose with them in family pictures when we've never felt a part of them in the first place.

Sometimes the only way we can save ourselves emotionally is never to return home and to form our own chosen families who prize information accessibility above all. Who wants to be told in so many ways (*Please stop lying that I was included—actions speak louder than words*) that we are not worthy of the effort of being included, especially after when we've worked so hard at learning to speak and lipread for *them*? And they couldn't be bothered to communicate with the same amount of effort that they expect us to extend?

Eventually we start to realize a startling fact: Hearing people are selfish. There's no way around that. They don't want to take the blame (*Well, we live in a hearing world*) for not trying harder to include us. To do so would require them to confront their own guilt and regret and all the ugly emotions that result, and to grapple with the hard questions of atonement and reparation. Such selfishness is a fine hallmark of hearing privilege.

Tell ...

So just what *is* Dinner Table Syndrome (DTS)?

I'LL TELL YOU LATER

Simply put, DTS encapsulates the plethora of negative and complicated feelings experienced by Deaf people when they are perpetually excluded from conversations by hearing people, causing them to feel isolated and often belittled, especially if those hearing people are the Deaf person's family. There is no question that DTS can be extremely psychologically and emotionally damaging. No one seems to make a point of warning hearing parents of Deaf babies about DTS.

That needs to change.

The four words that no hearing family member should *ever* tell a Deaf child are: "I'll tell you later."

The other four words, which are far more psychologically damaging, are: "I'm sorry I forgot."

After the first few times of anxiously wondering and waiting to know what a sister or an uncle had said that had been so funny, the Deaf child learns that they do not matter. Not really. They are to sit silently and pretend to enjoy the meal. The less they ask about what had been said, the better.

It is truly striking the way none of the hearing people at the table fail to pause and wonder why their Deaf family member aren't laughing. But oh, no matter: *No, really, she didn't say that! I thought Jack told her to pick green for his new car!—* These people may be already forgetting what had been so hilarious, but we Deaf people never forget the pain that burrows deep into our marrows. Aren't we supposed to be loved and treated equally to our own hearing siblings? We're already counting—not literally, but emotionally and psychologically. Throw in a few decades of this, and you *actually* have to wonder why we Deaf people can get so angry?

This anthology is a communal testimonial to the familial inclusion we Deaf people have longed to have while growing up with our hearing families. In these pages I want each one of us Deafies to acknowledge each other's feelings and experiences, and to know that we duly matter. Through an eclectic mix of poetry and prose, nineteen d/Deaf writers share what it was like to survive DTS and convey that experience in novel ways. Just like how many gay people have had to create their own "logical" (as opposed to biological families), Deaf people have had to redefine what *family* means to them. In doing so, they have survived.

If I can help increase a greater awareness of DTS through this anthology, awesome! It's my hope that future Deaf children will not have to go through the same psychological trauma of feeling so belittled among one's own hearing family. If hearing people expect Deaf people to change through the use of hearing assistance devices and speech therapy lessons, Deaf people *must* expect hearing people to change too! Hearing people *can* change; they just don't want to. (Selfish, selfish.)

We Deaf people are totally worthy of fulfilling meals with excellent company. We should not have to sit there and starve from so much loneliness while watching others feasting on so much laughter.

You ...

In a perfect world where hearing people are fully educated about the Deaf experience, this anthology would be completely unnecessary. We would find feelings of joy and warmth when we think about our own hearing families, even moreso if they signed or made sure that we were included in their conversations. We would know all the funny and jaw-dropping stories about our aunts and uncles and grandparents, and we could share them with each other each time we had a meal together. Through each gathering we add new stories about what happened to us that day. Each story becomes quilted into the folklore of our own identities—whether it be ethnic, religious, linguistic, and otherwise.

We inevitably feel jealous of our Deaf friends who grew up signing (*yay for full information accessibility!*) with their families, and the fact that they've experienced the full power of storytelling from generations past. (Of course, this is not to deny the fact that Deaf families can be just as dysfunctional as hearing families, but at least they had full language accessibility. And yes, some hearing families do actually make the effort to learn Sign, but they are rare.)

I've always said this about my own hearing family: They may have fully functional ears, but they do not know how to *listen*. They just babble and laugh away. I often have no clue what was so funny. They keep forgetting that I'm Deaf, as if that's a compliment to be seen as "normal," as one of them. Oh. Right. *Right.*

My best antidote to experiencing such pernicious pain is to attend any Deaf gathering and simply absorb how Deaf people interact with each other while eating. They do not hesitate to repeat anything if they weren't clear. That they may need to be repeat or rephrase themselves a few times doesn't matter. Deaf people are *very* sensitive about being fully included at any event, so making sure that others like them are just as included is just a matter of course. Everyone takes *turns*. That is like manna for my own eyes! It is one of the many beautiful things about Deaf culture: We may not have fully functional hearing, but we do know *how to listen*.

Deaf people are *my* true family. They do *understand*!

Later.

Last year I attended a casual party filled with hearing writers and artists in a large walkup apartment on the Upper West Side in New York City. While there, I met a hearing gay couple who lived nearby. They asked me what it was like to grow up Deaf with a hearing family. I didn't spare details. Then another couple sauntered into the room and began conversing with the first couple. They were clearly old friends.

But a most miraculous thing happened in that room. The older guy in the first couple—*how I really wish I could remember his name!*—looked at me and asked if I were following the conversation. I shook my head no. Unprompted, he quickly summarized in a quiet voice what the second couple had just said. He returned to the conversation, but he always looked at me every other moment and told me what had been said. I nearly couldn't lipread him, not because I couldn't follow him (he was actually very easy) but because I was fighting back my own tears. How was it possible for a total stranger who had no prior experience with Deaf people *totally* get me? If I hadn't believed before in the possibility of angels existing, he would've been Exhibit A. His intuitive compassion was truly extraordinary. If he hadn't been taken, I think I'd have fallen for him in a heartbeat. That he wasn't my physical type didn't matter. He had *genuine* compassion, an extremely rare quality that counts a lot more than just looks.

While I doubt that my own siblings would ever change to accommodate me, that stranger understood me in a way that I had so fervently wished to experience with my own hearing family. He gave me *hope* that other hearing people could be so intuitively compassionate.

So, if you are in a hearing family raising a Deaf child, please do *not* ever say, "I'll tell you later." *Unh-huh.*

And do not *ever* break that promise with "I'm sorry I forgot." *Oh no no no no no.* You absolutely can*not* do that.

Unless, of course, you want to orphan them and see them grow into adults you barely know, if at all.

By then they'll have left you because someone else did not break the promise of these four words: "I'll tell you *now.*"

Raymond Luczak
Minneapolis, Minnesota

Not Important

I was born and raised in Barre, Vermont, but I lived at the Deaf residential school in Brattleboro, a three-hour drive southeast of Barre. I went up to Barre on weekends and stayed with my family (I had seven siblings; I'm number five), but oddly enough, I'd always felt that I was only *visiting* them. I wasn't really living there. The Deaf school felt more like family to me than my own. I remember my oldest sister telling me once that every time I visited, my family had to "readjust" each time I showed up. Their eyes rolled as if displeased that I was there. "Readjust"? Their behavior made me feel like I shouldn't have been there. I don't know ....

I should mention that I didn't feel rejected by my family, but I did experience a lot of barriers. Most of my family outside of my siblings spoke French. (They were French-Canadians.) This meant I had to depend on my own family for translating between French and English. They simply didn't always want to do it for me. I wasn't important enough. It was frustrating because there were many times I wanted to know more about my family's history. Sometimes I got information; sometimes not. I saw how my family babbled quickly and excitedly, sharing the history I wanted so much to know. I missed out on all that. Like, for example, where did my mother's grandparents live? Did they live in the same house that they had inherited, or had they lived somewhere else before moving into that house? I never knew.

Most of my relatives are gone. So many of my aunts and uncles have died. There's only three left on my mother's side, and only one left on my father's side. (My father had come from a family of 17 children; my mother, 16 children.) Both large families: Think of all that rich history! I was really starving to learn all this stuff, but they mostly spoke French. Even one of my aunts asked my mother once why I couldn't speak French. "Is he stupid?" I felt like, "Why couldn't *they* speak English? Are they stupid too?" But my mother never said anything in my defense. That made me feel very small. I felt so disrespected as a Deaf person. (At that time, I wasn't blind, so I hadn't culturally identified as a DeafBlind person yet.) My family used a phrase that really bothered me: "deaf and dumb." It had historically meant "deaf and mute," but they spoke as if it meant "deaf and stupid." They believed that!

I've had two careers. I had a big and important job in the Theater Department at Gallaudet University. My family didn't believe that I could do that. Then I switched over to the Art Department where I ran the art gallery and the ceramics studio. And they still didn't believe that I could do that! I mean, that was the vibe I was getting from them. One of my aunts, one of my sisters, and my mother once flew down to D.C. and saw me at work. I showed my aunt and said, "Look over here! This is my work." I showed her the mechanism that rotated part of the set onstage for a play I was involved with, and I said, "I built this!" I showed her the machines that I used to build it. I did build the entire set onstage. I ran the tech stuff with my students. She paused and looked slack-jawed for a bit. She said, "Wow." Why is it so hard to believe that a Deaf person can do that?

I had two aunts and an uncle who were deafblind. I have no idea what my deafblind aunts did for a living—one was a housewife, and the other was unmarried. What did the unmarried deafblind aunt do for a living? Was she a nun? I don't think she was a full nun; she was a notch below that. Maybe she was a novitiate.

Now, my other deafblind aunt married a deaf man and had four children by him. I wanted to know more about these people and their lives, but again, my Canadian relatives spoke only French. I felt stuck. But I did learn that my deaf uncle died at the age of 99; he apparently worked hard, even mowing the lawn right up until his death. He was a very fit and mentally alert man. It was hard to communicate with him, but my Deaf brother—at the time he wasn't blind yet—was somehow able to interact with him. I still wanted to know more about my deaf uncle. Where did he study? Did they treat him as "deaf and dumb" like they'd treated me? To this day, I still have no idea!

Honestly, I've never felt a part of my hearing family. I'm not going to deny that. Yes, I was a Mama's boy. I really loved my mom, even though she had done some unforgivable things. I wasn't close to my father; I didn't like the way he treated me sometimes. For example, at the dinner table, he would use his fork to poke the back of my hand or my forearm to get my attention. He would tap his fork at a specific spot on his plate to tell me when he wanted me to lift a dish off the table and give it to him. He never spoke a word to me. He would poke me again when he wanted another dish and I'd have to bring it to him. He didn't like it when my Deaf brother and I, sitting directly opposite each other at the table, signed to each other during the meal. He tapped his fork on my hand and said, "I can do that, too." He made wild and exaggerated gestures that meant nothing. I felt so humiliated and yet ready to speak out loud with nonsensical babble, wanting to say, "I can do that, too," but I didn't have the nerve to talk back. I was so scared of him.

But I did refer to my reaction to my Deaf brother across the table. He burst out laughing.

Everyone looked at me. "What's so funny?"

I said nothing.

At the Deaf school, we all ate at round tables where we could see each other and sign. I never felt left out. That's why I felt they were my family. My time at the Deaf school—from 1964 to 1976 when I graduated from high school—were the best years of my life. I think it was because all of us were so lucky to have the *right* people, the *right* teachers, the *right* dorm supervisors—they were called "houseparents"—working there at the time. Many of them were new and freshly out of college, so they were very open to new ideas. They even signed! They ended up working there for anywhere from 20 to 40 years until they retired. I'm just very sad that the school was shut down in 2019. When a hearing school took over the campus, they allowed us to have the Austine School for the Deaf Museum so that all of us Deaf alumni could still visit and remember our history. I have so many wonderful memories of that place!

I grew up with this cousin of mine, and we were really good friends. Then I went away to college and she went away to have a military career. We lost touch for 35 to 40 years, but we finally reconnected through Facebook. She happened to be in the same town where my Deaf brother lived, and she wanted us to get together. I said, "Yes, I want to do that." I would go to her home for a light salad lunch. Then my oldest sister asked where I was going. She said she could drive me there and drop me off. Instead, she got out of the car and went right into our cousin's house. She took over any potential conversation between our cousin and me. I tried to talk directly with our cousin, but my sister kept saying, "He's wrong, he doesn't know what he's talking about." She kept gaslighting me. I started to see just how I never got the right information from my family because no one asked to make sure that I did. Why was I wrong? I mean, I was misunderstood. Simple as that. Yet during the few times I shared the truth during that conversation, my sister ignored the truth: "No, you're wrong." But I knew I was absolutely right.

One strange thing, though: If I met individually and alone with each of my siblings, my interactions with them were great. If I met with my brother, it was great. But when they all got together, I was not a part of them anymore. They were busy gibbering away. I'd ask, "What are you talking about?" They'd say, "I'll tell you later," and resume their gibbering. Yet, when I was one-on-one with my siblings, I could follow along and have a good time. But in their gatherings, I was not important.

Many of my friends at the Deaf school have experienced feeling unimportant among their own hearing families. For instance, my partner is the oldest of five children; he's the only one who is Deaf. His family treats him like a kid, and he's 50 years old! His mother forced him to clean the kitchen all the time when his siblings got together at their house. They'd give him dirty dishes, and he had to get straight to work. No one would help him. He has disowned his family for four years now. He refuses to talk with them anymore. His mother has repeatedly tried to contact him, but he's blocked her. At one point he did write her a letter of forgiveness, but just before he was about to send it, his mother did something—I don't remember what now—and right then and there he ripped up the letter.

I remember one thing in particular about my mother. When they discovered that I was deaf, the audiologist told my parents not to learn sign language because that would've prevented my ability to speak. Which is truly ridiculous! Duh. I was speaking just fine even with sign language. My mother expressed regret that she never learned how to sign even though she wanted to. Then on her deathbed, she expressed regrets about that a second time. I told her, "It's quite all right; don't worry."

Yes, I know that my parents did love me, but they were simply told the wrong things.

Many of my friends during our high school years shared their own struggles with their hearing families; back then we didn't have a name for that experience [Dinner Table Syndrome]. I did see a few hearing parents who learned sign language in order to communicate with their Deaf kids. That showed these Deaf offspring how important they were. But many hearing parents never learned how to sign.

I started to feel the full impact of DTS when I was in junior high school. I was starving for information. Up until then I simply focused on eating and piling more food onto my plate. I couldn't follow the conversation around the table, but I didn't care at the time. But once I was in junior high, I began to ask, "What are you laughing about? What are you talking about?"

They all said, "Later, later." I continued to sign discreetly with my Deaf brother right across the table. Sometimes he'd laugh at something I'd said, but he understood that laughing would've been considered an insult to our hearing family [because they didn't know what I'd said].

If I didn't have my Deaf brother, I can't imagine how my hearing family would treat me. I'd probably feel very alone. Maybe they'd treat me as a very precious kid. Or ignore me as always. It's hard to know.

Martha, my next-to-youngest sister, was the only one in my family who was genuinely motivated to learn sign language. In her job as a probational officer, she worked with Deaf clients from time to time. Then she and I would sign with each other. Sometimes she'd tell me things that she didn't want our family to know. That was kind of a neat reversal for me. Our family didn't know what *we* were talking about! They'd ask me what she'd said, and I'd say, "Nothing. Ask her." That's how I learned some of our family's history, like about my deafblind uncle who'd passed away. My sister was there when he died and went to his funeral. I couldn't be there; I was away at work. I happened to meet with her when I was on vacation, so I went to her house. She told me a sad story about our deafblind uncle.

Through her I learned that my father had a deafblind brother and that my mother had a hearing sighted sister named Eva. These cousins were dating. Eva stipulated that if he wanted to marry her, he would have to give up smoking and drinking. He refused. She said, "I can't marry you." (I should point out that my parents were also cousins.) I've always wondered if my hearing sighted aunt and deafblind uncle married, what would their children be like? Would they have deafblind children? Eva was one of my favorites, so I'd see her whenever I visited my grandmother. They lived together in a farmhouse. When my grandmother died, Eva inherited the house, but my deafblind uncle got the farm property. When Eva died, my uncle sold the farm and moved into her house. When he could no longer afford to maintain the house, he sold the house to Eva's son. So we're talking four generations in that house!

My grandfather not only built most of the furniture there, but also the house itself. That house is a favorite because it has so much history, and it is really a beautiful place. I mean, there are four bedrooms upstairs and one bedroom on the first floor where my grandparents slept. I always wondered how they could fit 17 children upstairs! What were their sleeping arrangements? I have no idea, but that's the sort of history I'm interested in learning. How did they live? But no one in my family really was willing to tell me, so ...

My third oldest brother is the worst of all my siblings. He always belittled me. He always made sure that I *knew* I was stupid. I hated visiting with him because if we had to shake hands, he would intentionally slither his hand about like a fish against my hand. After that, I simply stopped trying to shake his hand. If I arrived, I'd wave at him from a distance and stay away. If he ever went up to me, I'd move away and avoid him altogether.

He would make snide comments all the time, so I simply learned not to say anything. I didn't say much among my hearing family because I knew he would comment. I remember one time where I made beautiful pottery that I gave to my siblings for Christmas. When he got his bowls, he made a joke out of it. I said, "What? You don't like it? Let me take it back so I can give it to someone else who likes it." He said, "No, no. You misunderstood me." I said, "No, I don't think I misunderstood you. You were joking, which was hurtful. If you don't like it, say so. Give it to me." That was the first time I finally stood up to him.

That pottery was really hard work. It wasn't easy to create three nesting bowls so that all three could fit inside perfectly. *And* I used white clay, just like porcelain, which is much harder to deal with. The bowls did look beautiful, and I gave them to him. But he *had* to make a joke out of them. That experience made me feel like never making bowls for my siblings again. Of course, I did make more over the years, but there have been times when I'd like to have skipped my third oldest brother. But I've realized that if he wanted to be mean, that was just him. I wasn't going to be mean. I'm not a vindictive person.

One of the things that I learned fairly recently through Ancestry.com is that I have a half-brother. Apparently, years before he married my mother, my father had accidentally impregnated this woman. I should clarify: He chose to marry my mother, not that woman, who had to go to a convent for unwed mothers and have his baby there. This was considered a sin back in the 1950s. My half-brother never got to meet his biological parents; they both died before he learned who his birth parents were. With one exception—one of my brothers said that our father wouldn't do such a thing—he met with his half-siblings. It was truly remarkable how much he resembled our father.

The sad truth is that if I were to tell my siblings about my DTS experiences, I'm quite sure that they'd deny it. But then again, I avoid confrontations; I don't want to do that with my family. If they're not interested in me, I won't go up to Vermont and visit them as often the way I used to. I don't know when I'd go back up there to visit, but if my half-brother is going to be there, I will go and be there for him because he's as interested as I am in our shared family history. He'd been searching for his family, and now he wants to learn more about us. He would be asking a lot of the same questions I'd ask!

*

At our mother's funeral, Martha made sure that I was a part of it. This was because she had been the chair of a French-speaking festival a few times in my hometown. She demanded to have interpreters for me and my brother. It was a challenge, though, because there were so few interpreters who could understand French and translate into English via Sign. Turned out that there was indeed such a person, and I'd known her from Gallaudet. I was happily surprised. I was so impressed with her ability to deal with three languages at the same time! She'd listen to French music onstage, and she'd translate the lyrics into English and Sign. I don't know how she was able to do that! She was amazing.

Anyway, Martha always made sure that I had accessibility. It was important to her. She was the only one in our family who made me feel very important. She always made me a part of *her* family.

A Swiss Cheese Way of Life

Last year, I went to see a former student of mine—I'll call him R— graduate from high school. R was profoundly Deaf. His family was wonderful, but they didn't sign at all. The school and medical systems were such that they had never been strongly urged to, nor given the resources to learn. I was very fond of them, having been them through a lot with them during my teaching years. They'd taken public transportation to the graduation, and I offered to drive them home. When we got to their house, R's father and uncle were outside fixing a car. Seeing his nephew in a graduation gown, the uncle came to me and asked how to sign "congratulations." I showed him, and he went to R and signed a hearty "Congratulations" to him. R looked shocked, and tears sprung to his eyes. The two men hugged tightly. The uncle was a constant part of R's life since he was little, but I got the feeling it was the first and only time in 18 years that they'd had a meaningful exchange.

In fourth grade, R was transferred from the hearing, public school where I taught, to a Deaf school. There, he was placed in the Special Needs department. But what part of his intellectual delays were innate and what part were created by the family not signing? R was extremely well-behaved and hard-working, but had, when I met him, already missed five or six years of language.

What part for R and many like him, is actual intellectual disability and what part is handicap; the handicapping effect of being Deaf in a non-signing family?

One day when I was teaching, my students were lined up to go home, and my classroom aide excitedly told them that the following week was a vacation. I found most of them looking dismayed while the aide clapped happily. I grabbed a calendar, pointed to a day on it, and told them, "Look. She is right, it's vacation all next week. But on this day, we will all be back here together again!" Their faces brightened and they left, looking nervous but relieved. For them, vacation meant a week of no communication; of being dinner-tableized all day, every day.

School was a land of brain development, discussion, and inclusion, while "vacation" at home was a place of loneliness and being left out. Language Deprivation and Dinner Table Syndrome are closely intertwined; both occurring for the simple reason that families do not learn sign language.

Let me help you understand what language deprivation looks like. Imagine two six-year-olds on their first day of Kindergarten. One is hearing and one is Deaf. It is Monday, and each student had a birthday on the weekend. Let's say they are both on a school bus waiting to go home, and another child tells the bus driver about the birthdays. The driver, who is nicer than most and has time to spare that day, asks each kid what they did on their birthday. Did they get any gifts?

The hearing child has a thousand things to say. About her birthday party, her mom getting angry, their neighbor who didn't come because he had the flu, and so on. The Deaf child, though, doesn't understand the question. He nods happily when another child on the bus signs the word "birthday" to him, but when the child translates "The driver is asking *What did you do? Did you get presents?*" he has no response. He knows he had a birthday, and he has a lot to say about it, but he does not have the *language* with which to say it.

This will change rapidly if the child is surrounded at school by people who use ASL (or whatever the bona fide sign language of their country). In my class, it was as if ASL was a key that unlocked my student's brainpower and allowed information to flow freely in and out. It was glorious to witness, and it was an honor to use that key. My students went home ridiculously happily most days, looking like they'd won the lottery, simply because of language. They gathered new signed vocabulary all day and carried the new words/signs home with them like prizes, no matter how mundane they were. But at home, they couldn't share the source of their newfound joy with their parents. There, it was back to baby-talk.

In class we may have discussed the presidency, or multiplication, or seen a student from another class taken suddenly to the hospital, but at home rather than telling their parents the news, they had to revert to the home-made gestures their family used; *thumbs up, sleep, good boy.* It was a dystopian-level disconnect.

At some point in their lives, most Deaf people will meet families where the hearing parents and siblings *do* sign. Seeing this reveals to them that *not signing* was a *choice* their own parents made. A choice that had effectively barred them from one of the most essential aspects of being human; communicating with their own families. Which logically would make them question their self-worth.

And which is enraging.

I understand the enraged part because I am Deaf. I grew up in a hearing non-signing family, taught Deaf students from non-signing families for thirteen years, have many non-signing hearing friends, and am married to a hearing husband with minimal ASL skills. Intense frustration, despair or rage are not feelings one wants to have about their student's parents, friends or their own spouse. But they are valid and almost inevitable feelings in this situation.

As a teacher witnessing the communication breakdown between my students and their parents, I was shocked. Then I'd go home and experience it myself.

I'd make dinner, rally everyone to come eat, and realize I couldn't follow the conversation at all. Once a family dynamic like this has begun, it is extremely hard to reverse it.

If one interrupts their family dinner by saying, "Hey! I can't understand you! Please include me, this doesn't feel good," the family members have to recalibrate dramatically, changing from spoken English to a language they don't yet know, sacrificing their speedy conversation and their own need to have it. The Deaf person quickly looks, and feels, like the bad guy. It's hard because one doesn't want to ruin the natural flow of chat among others. But frustration is coursing through one's veins.

How to cope?

At age ten, I became suddenly Deaf (100% deaf in one ear and 95% deaf in the other). Having had a decade of absorbing a solid language foundation via spoken English before losing my hearing, Language Deprivation was not an issue for me personally. But from that point on, I too was left out; in was one-on-one conversations in a quiet room where I would do okay, especially with those I knew well. But all it took was a second person walking into the room and joining the chat that I'd be promptly ejected out of the conversation, no longer able to follow it.

In group situations I'd miss 95-100%.

As a child I was extremely outgoing and gregarious. I was so facially expressive that my dancer/theater director grandfather called me "the paper clown." As I got older, I loved bantering with strangers "the way some people love money," as I described it in my memoir *The Butterfly Cage*. When I became Deaf at age ten, I shrugged it off as being just another grand challenge to overcome and out-do by humor. But my parents were wracked with worry and guilt.

I didn't see why. I wasn't harmed or changed, and I didn't think it would change the core of who I am. But knowing how friendly I was, and how being Deaf would limit my social interactions, my parents weren't so sure.

It was, and continues to be, one of the most painful things I have ever experienced. The combination of being with loved ones and not being able to access their jokes, arguments, questions, and stories, is brutal. Missing out on their discussions of what to do later that day, only to be caught by surprise when they follow through with a plan you were not privy to. The odd sense, especially as an accomplished adult, of being infantilized in this way.

There are no bad people here. Instead, there are invisible differences between us; we are a universe apart while right next to each other. Apart not just in terms of communication but psychologically. Being Deaf is hard to believe; hard to imagine. And with those of us who are in-between Deaf and hearing; i.e., able to speak, and understand *some* things, *some* times, it is all the more confusing to others. They don't realize that it is totally situation-dependent and ever-changing. That the lack of comprehension can be a complete pain. That we can try to lipread so hard our eyes feel like they're bleeding, and still nothing makes sense. An hour earlier, in the backyard, they conversed with us easily, so it doesn't make sense to them that we are now at a total loss. When we are little, we don't have the wherewithal to explain it, nor do we totally understand it ourselves. And when we are older, it can be too late for people to change their established patterns.

My family used to eat dinner together. The dining room was cozy with a hanging lamp, the food was delicious, and conversation was lively and imaginative. But after becoming Deaf, I found the chatter going right over my head. I couldn't keep up, and realizing no one knew it, I felt stunningly alone. One day I suddenly blurted out, "I can't understand anything you're saying!" and bolted from the dining room up to my bedroom, slamming the door.

At one point I attended a big hearing high school where there was a Deaf program, in which nothing was being taught! It is just social time. Concerned, I met with a counselor and asked if I couild attend hearing classes part-time and the Deaf class, which was very relaxing, part-time. His answer? "No. You must pick one or the other." Next I asked, "If I switched to the hearing classes, can I have interpreters?" (It was my legal right, but I didn't realize that at the time. Neither did he.) Again, the answer was, "No. We don't do that."

I decided on the hearing classes, where I thought I might have a chance at education. But again I had underestimated how Deaf I was. In a Greek mythology class, I could not catch a single word in an hour of trying to lipread the teacher. But I did make a friend there. Somehow she had excellent grades but also had a habit of cutting classes. She would go through a hole in the metal fencing surrounding the campus, sit on a hill and smoke pot. I began joining her, because it helped to reduce my frustration of not hearing the teacher.

One day in my early twenties I attended a party where everyone was hearing. I held court in the kitchen, telling story after story to a group of listeners. By dominating the conversation like that I was able to "participate," and the crowd listening grew and seemed to enjoy it. When I left, I had a flicker of pride, but it quickly got submerged by a sense of emptiness, because I knew absolutely nothing about the other guests. I had not made any real connections, nor did I feel fulfilled.

What does it mean to be with—but also not be—with other human beings?

One day I rode my bike with a growing anticipation across Berkeley to my sister's house. Once there, I took in the atmosphere, food, discussions, arguments, jokes, howls of laughter. I suddenly realized I had been trying to understand, via lipreading, for an hour and had not caught more than three disconnected words. Visually, the conversations did not look lightweight, but only "mayonnaise," "San Francisco," and "pajamas" had emerged, clearly, from three different glistening mouths. I was struck forcefully by an intense sense of longing to understand who I was from observing my family members.

I felt a million miles away, despite the bodies surrounding me.

Depression began to set in.-

My older sister winked at me, laughing, sure she knew what I was thinking about what just said. It shocked me that she had no idea—or wanted no part of knowing—the deep funk I was sinking into. I felt encased in a bubble; hard, invisible plastic around me forming a sound barrier that no one could see, and no meaning could get through.

The alone-ness in the bubble was devastating.

I wondered why I was there; literally, why did I think this was going to go well?

And I felt fleetingly suicidal.

I began taking short story writing classes at college. I decided that someday I would follow my parents' footsteps and write a book. It would be about the hard of hearing experience. There were books about the deaf and there was a Deaf culture and community, I felt, but what about those living on the fringes? Where communication with hearing people was a constant ordeal, where one's ability to speak made everyone assume one could also hear, and where one wasn't yet a bona fide member of the Deaf community? What did it mean to be an Inbetweener whose numbers ranked in the millions, but who had no community? I'd write about how daily life for us was so characterized by holes and missing info that our thinking became like Swiss cheese. A world in which nothing was certain.

I loved Israeli folk dance, which involves many partner dances. I went often. Before the music started, I'd quickly tell my partner that I was Deaf and wouldn't be paying attention to them, but rather to the dancing. At the end of most dances, though, they'd look at me oddly. I'd realize that despite what I'd explained to them, they were chatting with me while we danced.

Once, on a trip to see my sister and her husband, we went on a long car ride. They were sitting in the front and talking. From the back seat, I couldn't understand them and gave up trying. I thought we were going to a restaurant to eat, so when they stopped at a 7-11, I stayed in the car. When they came back, they asked if I'd gotten food.

"I thought we were going to eat out," I said.

"No. We decided to get food here and have a picnic!" they said, exasperatedly. They didn't mean any harm; they just hadn't fathomed that I was 100% out of the loop of their discussion.

My date answers my questions in a large café with big echoey walls. He has a nice face, I thought. He seems to be a pretty happy person, laughs a lot, is self-effacing. But what the heck is he saying?

The more interested one is in other people; the more curious, the hungrier they are to understand what is being said. In other words there's an inverse relationship mathematically to the pain of missing out. If we don't care about what someone is saying, there's no problem. But if we do, it hurts. There is anger and conflict over it, while at its source was love; how much we love them and thus want to understand them.

Jump forward in time again. I have married this man I first met in the café, and we have two hearing daughters. I have not yet begun asking him to learn ASL, although I do after a few years. He tries, taking Level One twice, but refusing to do the homework or let me practice with him. Because I can speak and lipread, albeit with great difficulty, one on one, he doesn't feel signing is truly necessary. I learn this in a striking way when one day many years later my hearing aid has a problem. Not realizing this, I think I have gone completely Deaf. I text him, and he says, "Well, I guess I'm learning ASL then!"

Flash forward again. I was a mother in my forties, hosting a Thanksgiving meal at my home for friends and relatives. Suddenly I realized there was no need for me to sit at the table with them, and that it might be better if I didn't, given that I'd miss all the discussion.

I felt a bit insane for having hosted the meal under those circumstances. Why did I keep putting myself in these situations?

How do we not appear bitter in such circumstances? How can a hearing person understand it? My identity as a capital-Deaf person became more and more firm, over the course of the ten years I taught, but I remained stuck in a quagmire in my personal life.

Was I slow on the uptake? Yes.

But this is common. The understanding of how little conversation we can catch, and what might work better, comes to us in waves, levels, and grows in leaps when triggered by particularly memorable incidents.

When I finally got my teaching credentials, I quickly landed a job teaching at a mainstream (public) school near my home. I was to teach a Deaf K-3 class.

The first day I met my students. I was struck by their beautiful, shining, intelligent, cooperative, excited faces. They seemed incredibly hungry to learn.

"I'm happy to meet you!" I signed. "What's your name? How did you come here today, car, bus, or airplane?" I tried different questions, slowly, clearly, waiting patiently, and the children smiled broadly at me. But to my surprise, I got exactly zero answers. "How old are you?" I tried. Nothing. Finally I got a few names and ages. Names were spelled with odd and missing letters, ages were wildly inaccurate (unless there were a few 70-year-olds and one baby in the class).

I began to realize the kids didn't have a foundation of language. Their parents had not learned to sign and the school hadn't done much better.

Later that day, a fight almost broke out between two boys. One student was about to punch the other, who was cringing. I ran over and asked what was going on. No answer. I asked, "Are you angry?" to the one punching. He nodded. I had him sign, "I'm angry!" Surveying the situation, I asked if he was angry because the other boy was too close to him. He nodded. I signed, "I'm angry because I want more space. Please move." The boy copied me, and the other boy immediately moved.

Problem solved. Just like that!

And so began my ten-year-long deep dive into language deprivation, trying to understand how it happens, reverse it and teach academics at the same time.

The students had been exposed to Signing Exact English (SEE) signs from their preschool teacher, homemade signs from their families, and a smattering of Mexican signs, but otherwise had been inundated by spoken English and Spanish, which was about as meaningful to them as hieroglyphics. As a solution, they'd made up some signs, but their thinking skills remained extremely limited and foggy due to the constantly being left out of meaningful dialogue.

I began to energetically expose them to new signs, new words, new idioms, all in ASL, throughout the school day, trying to replace the made-up signs and SEE with the more impactful and accurate ASL. They rapidly soared in their new language, happiness, and academics. But their communication at home remained impenetrable.

I shared my home phone number freely and encouraged parents to call me. My hearing husband knew Spanish and could translate in a three-way phone call if they needed. They often did call. One parent asked me, via my husband, to explain to her child that the family was moving in a week. "We keep trying to pack his belongings up. Then he flips out and unpacks them," she explained. "But we can't explain to him that we are moving."

I could, and did, in less than three minutes the following day, using ASL and a quick sketch of two buildings. Another parent asked me to tell her daughter they had a dentist appointment the next day, so she'd pick her up early.

Basic everyday communication like this was missing within these families. But what about when it is less basic? When I was 14, I visited a Deaf friend at her home. Her brother and father asked me to come into another room for a moment. I did, and they explained, via voice, that that my friend's favorite uncle had died. Would I tell her please? I did, and she asked when? Six months ago, they said. She went ballistic. Who could blame her?

Yet still her family didn't learn to sign.

Imagine using only handmade gestures like the one for "eat" or "no" to discuss these issues with your beloved child as they march through life: birth, death, relationships, dreams, goals, mental health, and personal values.

Recently I saw a post on social media, where a teacher of the Deaf said she found her student was living with a hearing cousin the same age. The cousin showed up in the classroom one day, and the teacher asked what the two children liked to do together at home. "We don't do anything together because she can't understand me," the cousin said simply.

One day I found my students had absolutely no idea what boundaries they had a right to—when it came to physical contact between them and adults—since their otherwise protective, loving parents couldn't explain it to them. I taught a spontaneous fifteen-minute self-defense class where I had them practice and role-played—the fact that no one had the right to touch them if they didn't want it.

K, a fourth grader, fought off a rape in her home the next weekend.

She was hard of hearing and wore a hearing aid. But would she have understood me as fully, as deeply, as actionably, if I had been speaking, rather than signing, when I discussed boundaries? I am sure not. It felt odd, as a teacher, to tell my K-3 students about such a personal topic. But it is typical for teachers of the Deaf.

The families cannot and do not go deep into these topics like they do with their hearing children, without signing.

Would K have fought off the rape without that discussion? Based on the level of understanding my class demonstrated about boundaries a few days earlier, I strongly doubt it.

So why don't the parents learn ASL? First, they are not told to. They are busy, struggling for survival. If doctors, administrators, teachers, audiologists, and pediatricians, *all* required ASL from the parents; if they were given a free and convenient way to learn it, if they were not allowed to enroll their kids in school without committing to it, if they understood how it would impact their futures, early on, things might be different.

At every Individual Education Program (IEP) meeting, I explained passionately to the parents why they should learn to sign, especially for the profoundly Deaf students. Often, I'd get emotional and so would they. I'd offer to tutor them at any time, any place. I'd lend them materials, videos, whatever I could find. (Nowadays there are way better and more plentiful resources online.) I taught an ASL class at night, free of charge, I provided food there, and when I could, childcare. The parents came erratically.

One mother gave me a note via her child, asking me to send home something so she could learn signs. I immediately did. The girl was hard of hearing and was great at picking up the pronunciation of certain words, but when her hearing aid was off, she needed signs. However, at the next IEP, I asked the mother how the signing was going and she said, "I changed my mind. *My* daughter doesn't need sign after all. She is beginning to talk better now. She can understand me just fine." In this way, much as I was in my home life, the child was punished for her excellent coping skills.

Another parent said she would learn to sign if any of her family members would join her but her other kids were all busy teens and her husband had to work.

At what point will hearing people realize *their accountability* in communication? Because at that point, life would become dramatically better for Deaf people, of *all* ages. The positive trickle-down effect would be tremendous.

So, here is my grand plan to eliminate language deprivation. It's actually not that hard. If *all* children, not just Deaf and hard of hearing but *all* children, of *all* ages, in *all* public schools, learned ASL from an early age throughout school, embedded in the curriculum from K-12, the world would be drastically altered. There would be all kinds of benefits for the hearing kids—unrelated to deafness—and for the Deaf/hard of hearing kids, the whole landscape would change, since everyone, everywhere they went would be able to communicate easily, code-switching whenever they wanted or needed to.

Signing is not the only solution, although it is an extraordinary one, especially for developing young brains. But ensuring that the Deaf or hard of hearing person amongst you has full access can take many forms. During a family meal, one could plan things beforehand, remove visual obstacles, stop the conversation frequently and check the person is following, catch them up, use voice to text apps, use paper and pen, tell them if the topic has shifted. It is *ignoring* the issue that is a mistake.

I am no longer teaching, having retired early to write a book about everything I saw and learned while teaching. Watching my students navigate adulthood continues to inform me about how language deprivation is affecting them still (and quite profoundly.) Those that switched to a Deaf school (where everyone signed) have better thinking skills and are less isolated.

I am still married to the same man and last year had my first holiday ever that I could understand the conversation at. (I invited only Deaf/signing people.) It was glorious.

I recently have had to decline some amazing events that combined both writing and other vital interests of mine, because the attendees do not sign. I know how uncomfortable it would be to try constantly to lipread them, and they are not the type events where I can request an interpreter. I have finally begun to understand these situations don't work for me. My parents were not so wrong after all; by necessity I've become more introverted, and find myself hoping strangers don't try to talk to me.

Solutions like voice to text apps can work in a pinch, but for social situations they are extremely flawed and fallible. So what are my options? Find Deaf people to hang out with or make peace with self-isolating.

I find it fascinating that 95% of strangers I meet in public places say—when I tell them about the prevalence of, and reason for, language deprivation—that if they had a Deaf child they'd learn to sign immediately! How does this 95% figure compute with the *actual* number of those who do? I think school and medical professionals are squarely to blame here. Parents might think: eleven professionals have told us to get hearing devices and mainstream our kid so they'll "fit into the hearing world," while only *one* individual Deaf teacher said to learn ASL. Professionals must know what they're doing! Plus, my child seems fine. We get by okay.

It is a shockingly low bar, but, condoned by "professionals," getting by becomes the standard.

There is less need for Language Deprivation to exist these days since there are more free ways for parents to learn ASL online. But the thinking of hearing people is unchanged. If anything, the rise of devices like cochlear implants has made the problem worse than ever. Deaf people can and should lipread and learn to speak, they assert and assume, in order to fit better into the hearing world.

On social media once in a while I see amazing videos; for example there was one where a whole neighborhood came together weekly for an ASL class by a Deaf man. The inspiration for this was a two-year-old Deaf child who lived there as well, and yet the beauty of the weekly gatherings was multi-layered and far-reaching. And I have recently met parents of Deaf kids, who sign, as a family, even if their child can speak.

From my teaching years, there is one gorgeous occurrence. It is a parent, who is now fluent in ASL, having taken classes at a community college. My pride in her is tremendous. Like R's uncle did, the day his nephew graduated from high school, I wish her a hearty congratulations.

But in this woman's case, rather than being an anomaly—or the end— it is the *beginning*; of a potentially amazing career and new community for her, of knowing that she has done the right thing, as a parent.

In ASL, she has found the key and unlocked the door to magnificent, limitless and life-long communication.

Breaking Social Bonding

The name "Dinner Table Syndrome" (DTS) is something of a misnomer. Although it occurs most frequently within the core family at meals such as dinnertime, it arises during any large group gathering such as family reunions, Christmas, Passover seders, weddings, and the like. Many advocates for Deaf people often focus on the impacts to Deaf people in terms of missed opportunities for language acquisition and "incidental learning."[1] While this is certainly true and important, I would argue that a significant impact of DTS accrues to the development of social relationships and familial bonding.

Interestingly enough, before writing this piece, I attempted to conduct a search for professional literature on the topic of the role of communication in development of familial and social relationships, and I was unable to identify any that spoke to this topic. This is unfortunate, yet unsurprising, as Hearing people generally take it for granted that children are automatically and fully included within family activities by dint of their mere presence. In addition, while the effects of language deprivation can be seen quite early on in a child's development, the social/emotional impacts of DTS are cumulative and varying in how they manifest in the individual.

I'd like to emphasize that as with Language Deprivation, DTS and its effects does not arise solely in those with little to no auditory access to the world; it can also be seen in those who, by all outward appearances, would not be expected to experience these issues at all. To illustrate, I was born (at the very end of the great "Rubella Bulge" of the 1960s) Deaf to Hearing parents. I was the youngest of three boys. Upon my identification as Deaf around one and a half years old, my parents, as almost all did at the time, began an intensive program of speech and auditory training with the goal of raising me as "oral" with the ability to speak orally and comprehend oral speech by "lipreading" supported by utilizing my "residual hearing" through the use of hearing aids. As it happened, the amplification provided by the hearing aids brought my

---

1   "Incidental learning" describes learning by the child that takes place without explicit instruction through overhearing adult and other conversations or discussions regarding topics such as money management and medical matters as well as interpersonal relationships and feelings.

ability to perceive oral speech sounds mostly within the "Hearing" range, allowing me to develop the ability to produce extremely comprehensible (by outsiders) oral speech. In addition, I was reading independently by age four (my mother claimed I was correcting her spelling at five years old), which she attributed to some conjunction of the International Teaching Alphabet (a variation of the International Phonetic Alphabet used in my oral preschool program), regular viewing of *Sesame Street* (despite its lack of captions), and the fact I was interacting with the English-speaking world through oral speech as well as in writing. When my Oral preschool program began implementing "Total Communication," teaching signed English along with speech, my parents pulled me out of the program into a Hearing Kindergarten classroom full-time (after about a half-year trial period). Following this, I was fully mainstreamed in public school without any special service support other than regular speech therapy sessions and an occasional itinerant teacher pull-out to give me individual spelling tests (so I could lipread them instead of trying to lipread the regular teacher as she walked around the classroom) and for tutoring in math (which has always been my weakest subject). I remained in public school programs until the seventh grade and was always a top student in academic subjects (except for math).

Although by all outwards appearances I had achieved Hearing "normalcy," I was never "Hearing" and I always knew it. Due to the sensorineural[2] cause of my Deafness, although I was able to perceive a great deal in the way of *sounds*, when it came to the sounds of speech, I never developed any ability to *comprehend* these sounds without additional visual support, usually by lipreading. Without lipreading, oral speech sounds like gibberish, with maybe an occasional actual word caught here or there. To illustrate, I heard some of the refrain of a popular song by a well-known singer from the '80s as something like "BOBBY BARBIE DIE! Whoaaaa Oh! Ba me lay oh me kiyah ..." (I challenge you to figure out what this song is.[3])

In addition, I never developed the ability to geolocate any sound. Consequently, whether within the family or the classroom, I was at a distinct disadvantage in trying to keep up with group conversations and discussions. I have found that it can usually be fairly easy enough

---

2   Auditory nerve.
3   For those of you who are absolutely stumped, it's "The Longest Time" by Billy Joel.

to keep up in a one-on-one conversation (although certain people, like my middle brother, can be notoriously difficult to lipread). But every additional person who is added to the discussion increases the challenge of comprehending and following the discussion exponentially. It becomes more difficult to locate new speakers, and in sufficient time to establish the thread of their thoughts in order to follow them. Invariably, someone or other would talk while holding their hands over their mouths, looking away from me, mumbling, or some other lipreading-blocking behavior. Reminders to remove their hands or face me never took hold: In the space of five to ten minutes, these behaviors would inevitably be repeated. After a short amount of time, I would invariably find myself so far behind and at sea that it wasn't worthwhile to try to keep up. And of course "later" *never* comes!

Consequently I developed the habit of greeting arriving family members and responding to their perfunctory and *pro forma* questions, perhaps staying with the family for a few minutes for appearances' sake before making a hasty retreat to an unoccupied room where I could read a book (or later after the advent of closed captioning, watch TV). Meals were consumed as quickly as possible, and I would make my retreat at the earliest possible opportunity. My family's informal labeling of my behavior was that I was "antisocial." To the contrary, I was (and am) not antisocial: Indeed, as I lay on the sofa reading, hearing every burst of laughter from my family was a painful reminder of their casual, seemingly uncaring acceptance of my exclusion from participation within these events. I recently saw a meme that perfectly encapsulated my feelings and frustrations about the "antisocial" label: "I'm not antisocial; I'm deaf. It's not that I don't like or want to spend time with you, it's just that I can't understand what's being said around me." It's truly the classic double-bind situation: You're damned if you do, you're damned if you don't. Stay and be ostensibly "part of the group," but in reality you're entirely outside of it, or make your exclusion overt by leaving and getting criticized for it.

During one of my mother's attempts to exhort me into participation in these gatherings, to "just try harder" (How? Force my body to grow new ears or neurons within my auditory nerves or something?), she said something to the effect of "family gatherings are fun." My response (whether this was said aloud or only in my head, I don't recall now) was, "They're fun for *you*—for me, they're torture!" This was probably the last time the subject ever came up—at least in this way.

Entering as a teenager into the Deaf community rescued me from this life. I began to see what was possible—interacting with other people in a natural, instantaneous manner wherein I was not at the mercy and whims of other people to make me feel included. And yet, when I inevitably had to return home, the old wounds remained.

To protect myself psychologically, I developed a strategy of withholding by sharing less of my life with my family members, including my parents. They had proven that they would never understand or be able to overcome their entrenched audism. Since I had made it so easy for *them* to understand me by learning to use my voice in a comprehensible manner, they took this to mean that somehow, I was somehow able to understand them through auditory means, despite my repeated insistence and reminders that this was physically impossible for me. Therefore, why should I give myself emotionally to them when my access to them as people was limited by their own doing? I came to resist attending family gatherings, since this would mean extensive and expensive travel and time costs with no emotional or other benefit to myself. This emotional withdrawal and unresolved communicative issues created a certain level of tension with my parents, especially my mother and me. In the year after my father's passing, I attempted to try to get closer to my mother again, but after nearly a lifetime of unspoken and unresolved tensions, it was too late.

About fifteen years ago, my only uncle—my father's brother—unexpectedly passed away. By all accounts, Uncle Mitch was a sweet, decent man who endeared himself to most people who knew him. Yet, my wife, who is hearing, was shocked to see I took the news with all the emotional impact of learning that a celebrity from one's parents' generation had died: With a small shrug, I commented, "He was getting old." While my father was all torn up about it, and I did feel bad for him, Uncle Mitch was little more than a stranger to me—I had never had access to the jokes and stories that forged those emotional connections in others.

I know my story is unique to me, and yet as we can see throughout this book, my experience is shared by just about all Deaf people from Hearing families in a multitude of variations. I suspect that just as we are now learning the specific impacts of Language Deprivation on Deaf people at the individual as well as the community level, we will eventually find that DTS impacts all Deaf people at more than just the linguistic level—there is both an *individual* and a *collective* psychosocial cost to it that has an effect on ourselves and our relationships with Hearing people—especially those closest to us: our families.

Dreaming the Way Free

There's only one way to grin and bear it,
as the voices murmur round, one
story after another tumbles through
the space while I sit, watching each
word go, each face constrict with
laughter or tears—

I waver in the background, think of
the seashore, the way the waves crash
against the sand,

I dissolve here.

Is it an acceptable erasure
if I use this time to dream?

I imagine what I'll do the next day, or
how the world will look when my eyes
open in the morning.

> (Every person is an island; after all, I
> have my own trees and plants to tend.)

In a perfect world, I'd slip off my seat, slide
beneath their feet with the dogs to feel
their soft fur between my fingers, let them
lick the sides of my face as I crawl
along the length of the floor,
find the space at the end—

an opening, between an aunt's floral legging and an uncle's
suit pants, perfectly ironed, black as my dog's nose—

where I can slip out, squeeze through

the back door, feel the wind on my face,
follow my dog to her favorite tree, stretch out,
dream with the sky.

An Interpreter Would Try

I'm not sure how many times
I can watch the story play out
through their eyes, the arch of their necks,
gasps they make as they tell a special part—

Not even the best interpreter could replicate
the way a grandmother chides her grandchild,
the pinch she gives their cheeks
at just the right line.

An interpreter would try to mimic
their bodies as well as their words, they'd try
with the effort of a runner near the finish line—
racing to get across, their hands
flickering wildly in ways only
the deaf person knows couldn't be right—

(we've grown up with these people, after all)

But there's no interpreter
at the family dinner table,
no one to attempt such a feat.

I wait for someone to explain, but the story
has already lost its spontaneity, the words
have lost their humor, the collective moment
passed—

KRIS RINGMAN

One Breath to the Next

Sometimes when they are speaking so loud
unclear hands down mouths filled with food
hands in front of mouths faces turned away
murmurings into another's ear their heads
nod as they laugh arms up in the way again
can't see the angles keep shifting as they turn

I lose sense of myself—

take a deep breath—

I melt into the wood skin of my chair,
how well I come to know its
curves as I slide down
across the floor, I send
tendrils of myself
up the sides of
legs.

I feel one woman's ache, another's
dismay,
a man's joy, another's
dream—
someone's complex explanation of something
they adore—
people stare at the same place in the air
between them, as if they all see something
I can't see at all—
I feel questions, misunderstandings,
blurred desires—

I feel everything
when I can't hear it,
none of it solid held up

by the fingers of a story
given context given a shape
at all for me to grasp an edge.

It burns
like brushing against
the stinging nettle as you
rush down a trail, the forest
a green blur around you
like their mouths.

I feel every tremble
in the room, even as they hide
their hands under the table, it is
my space down here, another level
of existing in the room where I feel
every heart beat beneath the texture
of each person's shirt fabric, mostly soft
porous knits, buttons of shiny plastic.

I want to place my hand on
their chests, I want to help, beg them
tell me a story I can follow, tell me
anything at all, I am here.

I disappear I am here
not here inside myself
inside you always
between.

Last Rites Are Never What You Expect

The worst part
is the words I can't catch:

My husband and his cousin's slow deliberations, what to eat, how much
food to make for a gathering, the color of the
tomatoes, or their taste in our mouths.

Without these words, there's no path to lead me through
the routes of their memory. The dead brother-in-law
I never met.

But they are still here and so am I. When the words
fall around me, I trip, I stumble,
I roll away under a couch with the dust, closer to the dead.

Deaf. Dead.
            I once had an interpreter mix up these words.

Like the small talk we make in the wake of death,
every lost word carries a world of meaning
in the blur it makes across the room—these sentiments
I can't follow streak like ghosts sucked back into the corners of the
        room
where the dust of everything said and unsaid
hovers.

I feel no different from the ashes, scattered,
dirty, ashamed of my own radiation. Each question
I answer wrongly. This intensity I cannot push down—I hide
as if I am made of the same
toxic powder,

the same crushed bones they packed in a box
and shipped away. I shouldn't

be touched. I hide, because
there is too much nuance—
how can I comfort them if I can't
understand what they're saying?

How can I participate
in anyone's death—
        in anyone's life?

Pieces of the Ceiling Falling Down Around Me

Most deaf people I met later in life—the ones like me, from Hearing families—they all said the same thing: *Nobody ever told them anything.* They'd sit there through every meal; breakfast, lunch, and dinner, watching everyone yap away. One guy said he felt like the family dog, that he might as well have not even been there. His real place was under the table. Like a good dog, well-trained. Patiently waiting for whatever scrap some Hearing person might flick off the plate.

For what it's worth, though, Anne wasn't like that. She learned to sign almost as soon as I did.

For what that's worth.

"She's your older sister, you said?"
    "My oldest sister. By like seven years."
    "This is a large family? You have many siblings?"
    "Yeah. Two brothers, two sisters. In that order. Then me. I'm the baby."
    "Anne is the middle child?"
    "Yes."
    "And the only one in your family who signs?"
    "Yes."
    "I'm sorry. I just find that heartbreaking."
    "It's common."
    "You have a deaf brother as well, though?"
    "Scott. He never went to a school for the deaf. He speaks. Better than I do."
    "That's ... very interesting. Did he ..."
    "Doc. I don't want to talk about him."
    "Okay."
    "It's too fucking much."
    "Okay."
    "I don't know why people do what they do. My parents ..."
    "It's okay."
    "I guess my parents didn't see that as an option for him. Or maybe schools for the deaf weren't as popular in the sixties. When he was a kid."

"Okay."

"I didn't learn to sign until I was thirteen. That was in '83. I don't know what anyone's plan was for me. I don't ... my Mom ..."

"Dan."

"I don't know."

"Dan. I'm sorry. I interrupted you. I shouldn't have done that. I'm sorry."

"I don't know what to tell you."

"Talk about Anne."

It is 1977. I am seven. Anne is fourteen. I'm screaming at her because Star Wars is playing at the movie theater. Actually, the most accurate way to say this is I am Daniel Tallerman, fifty-four years old in the year 2024, standing in the corner of my childhood home, like the Ghost of Christmas Past, watching my seven-year-old self scream at her while simultaneously remembering myself screaming at her. If I *only* remember, without making myself go there, into the memory, my mind will eventually push things away, and then I *can't* remember. So I've trained myself to go into the memory and *stay*. In those moments. Really stay.

The carpet of the living room is red. The tiles of the kitchen floor are light lime green. The countertops are glaring orange. Our television is the size of a steamer trunk.

There is no consoling my younger self. Mom is screaming at Anne too. But how is she supposed to take me to see it? She was born in '63. She can't even drive.

Anne screams back. My younger self screams again. I remember only that the previews for the movie had shown up on the TV. I'd never seen anything like that before. Not a space battle, not an X-Wing, not a preview. I *had* to see it.

Finally, Anne runs out of the room. My present-day self wants to follow her, tell her that of course this isn't fair, it's not her problem. But it doesn't work like that. I can only see what I once saw. I can only go where I once went.

But I see so much more now than I did then.

She was only fourteen years old.

What could anyone have possibly expected her to do?

"Do these memories bother you a lot? Do they wake you up? Take up space during the day?"

"They used to."

"Not anymore?"

"It's a different problem now."

"Explain."

"When they woke me up, when I couldn't get back to sleep. I knew they were memories. If they weren't memories ... I wouldn't have remembered them. I knew they weren't dreams. Stuff my mind was making up."

"But now ... you can't tell?"

"Not exactly. I still know they're memories."

"But?"

"They don't feel like memories."

Anne ... has to be over sixteen. She can drive now. She has a Firebird Pontiac. She's still in high school, though, making it somewhere between 1978 and 1981. She has just come home, late at night, drunk. Our father is drunk, too. My older self watches my younger self as he watches them from the stairs. Anne's flannel shirt is brown, her high school letterman's jacket is red and tan. Dad has her by both collars, and is pushing her into the dining room table. She punches him in the ear, above the eye. Above the eye again. His skin is brown, weatherbeaten, his jean jacket is blue. His blood is red.

She punches him again. He lets go.

My younger self is rooted to the spot. I try to reach out to him, so he will know I'm here. But I can't touch anything or say anything. That's not the way it works.

"Dan. You're safe here.

Dan.

Daniel."

Only two good memories of Anne come to mind from my younger years. The first: It's early summer, 1985. I am fifteen. I'm at football training camp at the Wisconsin School for the Deaf. I've been going there for a year. My girlfriend from back home broke up with me two weeks ago. A letter arrives from Anne. I haven't seen Anne in years. In 1985, she was twenty-two. Long gone.

"What's it like in Platteville?" I asked her once. Right after she moved. Platteville was way west of Madison, where she went to tech school after she graduated.

"*A hell of a lot better than it is around here,*" she spat, and then I didn't see her anymore.

She came home that weekend to look for some financial aid papers but couldn't find them. Everything was always such a scattered mess. She was ready to cry, but Anne never cries, or at least she never lets you see this. Dad would be home soon and I could tell she wanted to be gone before that happened. He made everything worse. I felt bad for her.

I guess she took my expression the wrong way, and thought I was mocking her. She threw a bottle of aspirin at my chest. It bounced off, hit the floor. She had a *bad* temper. Whenever she fouled out in basketball games, she'd scream at herself, the ref, the players, and storm off the court. Hide her head under a towel and shake on the bench. Only her teammates could touch her. The Coach was a man. He would not go near her.

I try to read over my younger self's shoulder. *You need to hang in there*, it says (but I'm working from memory now—I can't actually make out the words). *There are more fish in the sea. You'll find someone.*

I remember thinking it was a nice letter. Not something that she had to write, like a birthday card to one of the Aunts. I guess Mom told her I was really shook up.

The second good memory: dancing with her at our sister Sue's first wedding. I have on a black tux and a purple bow tie. She has a purple bridesmaids dress that looks out of place on her, since she rarely wears dresses. The B-52s are playing "Love Shack." I clap, do a spin. She copies, laughs.

It's 1990. I am twenty years old. She is twenty-seven.

"*But you lived with her.*"

"*For a bit, yeah. In California. After college.*"

"But you don't ... remember much of her?"

"I remember her. I just ... by the time I more easily remember her, I was in my early twenties. I lived in California from like '93-'95. So I was a young man by then. I just don't remember her much from before that, when I was a kid. Just flashes. She was gone before I was out of grade school. She was in California before I graduated from high school."

"Okay."

"Dad threw her out."

"Why?"

"They hated each other. He was nuts."

"I see."

"Big time boozehound. Anne was a pain in the ass, though. Constantly partying. Disobedient. Rebellious. Even I could see that, young as I was. Our sister Sue became the same way for a while. But not as bad. She was nicer. Ended up marrying an alcoholic prick during her first marriage, but she wasn't as bad. She was like my Mom."

"Like your Mom?"

"Nicer. More rebellious than Mom but nicer than Anne. Our Mom was too nice. It gets you in just as much trouble."

"Anne wasn't nice?"

"Anne was like our Dad."

"Dan. Something to tell you." We're standing in Sue's kitchen. It's 1993. Anne is clearly nervous. More nervous than I've ever seen her. Her hands shake as she signs. This is the first time I've ever seen her sign. She's good at it, too. I'm surprised.

Our sister Sue has discreetly faded to the backdrop to play with JoAnna, who, at just over two years old, is already scampering around the living room at top speed. I'll miss playing with her, and the way she climbs out of her crib when I come home from the night shift at the factory, every single stuffed animal she owns scooped up in her tiny arms, giggling 'Unca Danna, Unca Danna' over and over until I pick her up and put her back to sleep. Sue is pregnant again. She's always tired. You can tell she's glad, though she doesn't say this directly, that I'm moving out and becoming someone else's problem. Likewise, I'm glad to be moving out and heading for California in a few weeks. I'm sick of

Broan Manufacturing. I'm sick of Wisconsin winters and freezing my ass off on the loading bay. I have my degree in English. I want to use it.

Go West, Young Man.

"Shoot," I say. Hoping to God Anne wasn't backing out of our agreement. There's no way I can afford a Los Angeles rent for long on the meager savings I've built up so far.

"When you come to live with Sarah and I. You remember Sarah, right? From last Christmas?"

"Sure."

Anne sighs. "She's not just my roommate."

I don't understand at first. I'm young. Twenty-three years old.

"She's ... more than that."

"She's a good friend?"

"... Yes."

"I'm not gonna make a move on her or anything, Anne."

Her eyes blazed. "She wouldn't *let* you make a move on her!" she snapped.

I understood, then.

"She's my girlfriend."

"Oh."

"*Yeah.*"

"I didn't know."

"I never told you."

"Okay." The trick to calming down Anne is to not react the way our Dad would. I remember getting earrings when I was twenty. The first thing he snarled: "*You ain't gay, are ya?*" Pretty much what he says about everything.

Suddenly, *everything* about Anne makes a lot more sense.

"So," she says.

"It's not a problem for me."

"I don't give a fuck if it's a problem for you."

I sigh. Not just my younger self, either. My present self, watching from the corner, breathes in deeply right along with him. She's *always* like this. Has always *been* like this.

"Anne," I say. "It's not a *problem*."

She looks at me. Decides I mean it. Nods.

"Is this why Dad ... ?"

"What."
"Is this? You know."
"No. He doesn't know."
"Okay."
"He's not *gonna* know."
Is this why he threw you out, I want to ask.
But Anne has already walked away.

"Why did he kick her out? Did you ever find out?"
"No. She hated men. Dad. Scott. We had this neighbor, a farmhand. Fucking hated him. Every guy she saw. Since she was a kid."
"I ... see."
"Through some miracle she got a boyfriend for a week in high school. Ended up telling him off outside the front door. Really getting in his face. Aggressive. Ready to hit him."
"It sounds like she was dealing with significant trauma."
"I guess."
"But I can't diagnose her when she's not here, Dan. I can only go on your impressions."
"I can't diagnose her either."

My later memories are clearer, but no less confusing. The same mix of good and bad.

It's 1993. I am twenty-three years old. Anne is thirty. We're at a party in L.A. Standing by someone's pool. Hearing people everywhere, talking, talking. I end up on a swing, suspended from a nearby tree, dangling my feet in the water. Some girl comes up. She's closer to Anne's age, but cute. She signs a little. We make do. She wants to know what it's like to be deaf.

I start telling her. It's an animated discussion, probably too loud.

After a bit, Anne comes up. Motions for me to come over. She has the Big Sister Expression on her face. Don't get the idea this will be a conversation of equal adults.

"People don't want to hear about your problems," she signs. She doesn't have to finish up with "shut it" or "knock it off." As much as you can hiss in sign language, Anne's the resident expert.

Another memory, months later: Anne has gotten me a night shift job at the special effects company where she used to work, and that pays alright. But I also found my own job, a daytime job as a tutor at Cal State University-Northridge. Ann seems strangely impressed, yet also angry about this. I don't care. It means I can move out of her house, and I do, right into one of the CSUN dorms on Nordhoff, even though I'm not a student (nobody asked). It's a real shoebox studio kind of place; with barely enough space for a foldout couch. But add in a television stand so I can put my feet up, and boom. *Home.*

My present self watches my younger self walk through the door to his first night of living entirely on his own. His eyes light up as he sees boxes upon boxes stuffed with things Anne and Sarah have either bought for him or given to him: a new television, dishes and plates and pans, blankets, sheets, everything he'd need. They even brought food and put it in the fridge. He calls them up on his TTY, placing the phone in the cradle.

THANK YOU, he types. GA.

ALL GOOD, they reply.

She even buys him a car. A used Toyota. "You gotta pay me back, though," she says, days later. "I'm keeping a list." From the background, Sarah smiles. Anne is softer with her around.

A good start to being in California.

"It didn't stay that way?"

January 24th, 1994. I am twenty-four.

Something hits my head. Softly. Gravel. Marbles?

I awake in pitch blackness. This is what immediately alarms me the most. The apartment is never that dark, even after sundown. The streetlights shine through the window, at least partially, even with the blinds closed. I always have the television on to keep myself company. A small night light is plugged into the wall socket in the bathroom so I don't have to flip on the switch for the glaring overhead light in the middle of the night.

But now? Nothing. Utter darkness.

The floor suddenly heaves, a ship on a storming ocean. I'm bucked from the couch and go flying into the darkness, slamming into something cold, metallic. It tips forward, pushing me into the floor.

Cold tile against my face. Not carpeting. *This is the kitchen. I'm in my kitchen.* A good five feet from the couch.

The room heaves again, followed by a rumbling that feels like a tank backing over the room, like a battleship dropped on the whole goddamned building. A mountain.

I'm young, I'm from Wisconsin. I don't understand.

All I can do is feel around for clothing, shoes, my jean jacket. All the while, pieces of the ceiling are sprinkling down on my head. By now I've figured it out. *Earthquake.* Eventually I see a flashlight beam under the crack of my front door. Someone pushes on it and gets a hand through. I see that my refrigerator has tipped over, blocking it. I tell the person to wait, *stay there!* and push the fridge upright again. We get the door open wide enough for me to squirm out.

The guy holding the light gestures down the hallway. Students are running past me in twos and threes, feeling their way along the wall towards the stairwell. Someone grabs my hand-a man or a woman, I don't know-and we each pull each other along.

Moments later, we emerged into the most beautiful starlit sky I have ever seen. A West Coast sky devoid of light pollution. The dorm is just across the street from a huge athletic field. We all run for it. Whoever is holding onto me lets go and is immediately sucked into the crowd. The ground heaves again and we all go sprawling. I slam face first into the pavement, scraping my forehead. I get up and stumble forward again. Eventually, I make it across the street to the grass.

All around, people are screaming, though I don't know this until the flashlight beams catch their faces. They are running towards me from the parking structure down the road where my car is parked. I can ... feel ... an ominous rumble, some horrible noise from all around, an infrasonic grating. Trees shake as if seized by a giant hand.

Giant fireballs rise up in the distance, at the opposite end of the field. More screaming. People run to get away from the rocking streetlights. My friend Gretchen lives near one of the fireballs. We just had a date.

Dinner at my apartment. Spaghetti and biscuits, the kind that come as dough balls in a pressurized cylinder. One blew out of the tube when I opened it, hitting the wall above the stove and sticking to it. I laughed. The heat would kill any germs when I baked it. What she didn't know wouldn't hurt her.

I learn later, in the smoky dawn of the sunrise, that her apartment building burnt down. Red Cross trucks are everywhere. We can't go back into our apartments. My sweatpants are on inside out, I have on two different shoes. No shirt, just my jean jacket.

The parking garage up the street has folded in on itself. And the Toyota Anne bought for me.

"*Jesus.*"

"*I was three blocks from the epicenter. It was a 6.7.*"

"*Did Anne and Sarah get hit?*"

"*They were ten miles out. Wasn't as bad. A bottle of wine fell off their fridge. Got stuck behind it when the fridge tipped back. Ended up punching the bottle through the wall. Didn't break the bottle. Just punched a hole.*"

"*Bizarre.*"

"*It's gotta be a metaphor.*"

"*The wine bottle?*"

"*The whole thing.*"

There's a middle to this story, but I don't get it, myself, so I can't tell it well. That's Dinner Table Syndrome for you. Bits and pieces you try to string together. Beyond that? You can always try asking someone to fill you in.

I'm sure they'll get around to it eventually.

1995. I'm about to move back to Milwaukee. I can't handle earthquakes. Anne isn't sad to see me go. Half of my stuff still isn't packed. Meredith from work shows up two hours early for the party, and my college roommate Bob has just flown out. He and I will take a drive-away back home tomorrow. Anne can barely keep herself together, telling me to hurry up and get everything packed so she won't end up having to do it. But Meredith's hand keeps brushing against my arm all night, and after the party, and nearly a whole bottle of tequila later, we end up fucking on the floor of the spare bedroom that Bob and I are sharing for the night. He hears everything, and says the next morning that I breathe like a locomotive. Anne is pissed, but makes us all breakfast, and after a curt hug from her and Sarah both, we're on our way.

1996. I fly back out for a weekend. I've earned enough flight points for a freebie trip. Meredith is history. Anne is mowing the lawn while I sit by the pool. She hits a snag somewhere, a stick or a rock or something, and yanks the mower back so viciously it jerks entirely off the ground. She stands there for a second, shoulders trembling, not letting us see her face, then carries on as if nothing has happened. Sarah pointedly looks away. I get the strong message: Don't fly out here anymore. So I don't.

1998. Anne visits Milwaukee with the special effects crew for some movie she's working on. Do I want to meet her? We meet on Water Street, near the fancy downtown bars. The crew seems excited, catching onto the vibe of the place. I offer to show them around. The Safehouse is just a couple of blocks over, right along the river ...

"I don't need a tour," Anne snaps.

I have no idea where this blast of fury comes from. Even one of the crew people who overhears is taken aback.

I don't give them a tour.

1999. I'm getting married. Anne and Sarah have broken up by this time. Something about Anne working all the time. I learned via Mom that she worked so hard one night she put herself in the ER with exhaustion. It was too much for Sarah, I guess.

Anne sits there sullenly, all through the dance, but it's a polka band, so it's hard to blame her. What can I say? Marie's family is big on polka bands. I'd gone completely deaf a year earlier and didn't care what music we had. It's not like we could afford Guns-N-Roses.

You'd figure that if I don't care, Anne shouldn't care. But Anne *does* care. She cares very much. You see this in her contempt, the way she all but hugs herself without hugging herself, her body a protective armored shell shielding someone deep inside, far beneath and far away. Believe it or not, I feel closer to her at this moment than I have in years. But Marie grabs my hand, pulling me back out onto the floor. Half our friends are completely smashed, and smashed is when you dance best, deaf or no. So fuck Anne. It can't always be about her.

2002. She got married. No word or invite to Marie and I. We're out in DC now. It's just after 9/11. We're both a few years into new jobs. We aren't thinking about her. Mom sent pictures and that's how we found out. Even Dad wasn't invited. I don't even know her new partner's name, since Mom doesn't mention it in her letter. I learn what it is later: Molly.

They have two children over the next few years. I don't hear about either birth until well after the fact, and I don't hear about them from Anne.

2010. Three years after our son is born. Marie learns through Facebook that Anne and Molly are traveling through Virginia. Less than an hour away from our house. We send Molly a message via Facebook Messenger: *Hey! Why not stop by on your way down through the state!* They reply: *Okay, we'll try!* And they do come by and stay for a night. We meet their kids; they meet our son. But it's awkward.

If we hadn't seen Molly's Facebook post, we would never have even known they were on the East Coast.

"That must have felt confusing."

"It was insidious, the distance. Damage done before you realized it."

"Did you see her again?"

"Off and on. More of the same thing. Push, pull, push. It got really bad, though, at the nursing home."

"When your father died?"

"Yeah. Well, no. He didn't die right away. He had a heart attack. He actually died many months later. But we all flew in that weekend. To say goodbye. Including JoAnna."

"This is your niece?"

"Sue's second daughter. Her middle child."

"The one who went deaf suddenly?"

"Almost overnight. Just out of college. She was Hearing all her life. Then had trouble. She thought it was earwax, at first. But no. Went to her ENT. Surprise, not earwax. It was a severe loss."

"That must have been quite difficult for her to accept."

"Deafness is a genetic time bomb in my family. It hit Scott and I when we were kids. Showed up later for her."

"And this all connects back to Anne?"

"Everything is about Anne."

"How so?"
"When it stops being about Anne? Trust me. Anne will let you know."

Sue won't come into Dad's hospital room with us. From what I can get from Anne, who is exhausted and doesn't want to interpret *every last little fucking thing*, Dad had a Do Not Resuscitate order signed and sealed at the nursing home. But he held on, and begged Sue to keep him alive so we could all fly in, and he could see us one last time. Dad's doctor wasn't happy about the situation and apparently yelled at Sue, telling her a DNR order was a DNR order, and it was a waste of time and resources to have him shipped to Madison. By this time the hospital had provided me with an official interpreter, so I later corner him in the hallway and tell him that if a patient changes his mind about a DNR order, a doctor says "Okay." And that's it—that's his place. Otherwise it's murder. So he should apologize to Sue, and stop being an asshole.

He says he'll apologize.

Anne watches this exchange in irate silence. Dad is stable for now. Anne and David, Sue's second husband, decide to take Sue out for brunch. I have to go with them. I have no vehicle.

I already ate at the Madison airport while waiting for Sue to pick me up. Egg, sausage, and cheese in a roll. I'm still on East Coast time. I was hungry then, I'm not now.

Pay attention. These details are important.

The family dog eats on command.

"You mentioned that Sue was already stressed out?"
"Yeah."
"In addition to what had just happened with your father?"
"She was mad at me."
"Why?"
"Because of what I said to JoAnna."
"JoAnna texted, you said?"
"At first, she just wanted to know about practical things. Where to buy a vibrating alarm clock, flashing lights for the doorbell. Speech to text apps. There was this guy at her workplace who kept sneaking up

behind her and scaring her, knowing she was deaf. She hated that shit. I hate that shit. I told her to get a mirror and put it on her desk so she could see who was behind her."

"Okay."

"But we got deeper into it, and I also said stuff like, she had to prepare herself mentally. Because there's a lot of things Hearing people won't be able to understand. Not even her Mom. They just can't. No more than any of us know what it's like to be blind just because we close our eyes for fifteen seconds and grope around in the dark. We can open them again. That's not the same as knowing. As being stuck with something."

"And Sue … didn't appreciate this comment?"

"She yelled at me. Said she's not like our Mom and Dad, that she intended to be there for JoAnna. And that JoAnna wouldn't ever go through the isolation that Scott and I did."

"She told Anne about this conversation?"

"Of course she did."

"I see."

"Strength in numbers."

We get to the restaurant. The four of us crowd into a booth. David. Sue. Anne. Me. Sue's eyes are still damp and red from her time alone in the truck, but she sucks it up and smiles for the waitress. There's a lot of Mom in her.

"I don't want anything," I tell the waitress. "Maybe just water?"

"Sure thing," she says, and finishes taking everyone else's order. As soon as she's gone, Anne looks at me. Once again, that Big Sister expression.

"Say 'please,'" she signs, disgusted.

I'm caught totally off guard. "What?" I sign back. Sue and David are oblivious. Anne shakes her head, and looks away.

Eventually the waitress comes back with our drinks, and asks what everyone wants to eat.

"I don't really want anything," I tell her. To which she mumbles something that I can't catch. I look reflexively at Anne, the only one who can interpret.

"Do you want popcorn?" Anne signs, glaring at me.

I get the feeling the waitress won't go away unless I order something. I smile, and give her a thumbs up. "Sure."

The waitress leaves. Anne is disgusted anew. "'*Thank you*,'" she signs, emphasizing the phrase. Because I'm too stupid to remember my manners on my own, see? And must be taught: *Sit. Stay. Speak*. '*Thank you.*'

"Are you fucking putting me on?" I ask her. And look at her steadily. Until she shuts up.

"Lots of tension."

"Yes."

"Your father was transferred out of Madison?"

"Back to the nursing home near Mom's house, yeah. We went to see him that night."

They have Dad in a large padded wheelchair. His body is held in place by a loose strap. Three separate IV bags hang from the drip stand behind him. Serious stuff. His skin is pasty and gray. But he's alive and alert.

Mom, Anne, Sue, and the Aunts are seated in a semi-circle around him, looking through boxes of old photos, selecting some for a giant photo album. Scott is watching football on television. JoAnna is scrolling through her phone. Dad seems more interested in the game than he is in the photos, but that's not saying a lot.

The Packers are way ahead. I lose interest, and start digging instead through one of the boxes of photos.

Pretty soon a really good one of Dad turns up. In this really sharp blue graduation suit. He was probably eighteen. Thin. Vibrant. Healthy. Everything in front of him. I totally bought into his smile.

I take out my phone to take a picture of the photo, since I know nobody will ever give me any of these.

I find another one: him in his Army uniform. I try to snap a pic. But my phone dies.

I find another one. A wedding photo of him and Mom.

"Anne," I sign, getting her attention. "Let me borrow your phone."

Puzzled, she hands it over. I snap a new pic, intending to send it to myself. But her phone's camera has the flash turned on. As soon as I press the button, a flare of brilliant light blinds nearly everyone in the room.

"Sorry," I mutter, and turn it off. I find new photos, snap pics of them, and send them to myself.

Anne grabs the phone out of my hand. "Do you have to do that *now*?" she signs, aghast. I have no idea why she's so worked up. Nobody else is looking at me. Or at her, for that matter. The Aunts go chattering on. Dad is completely out of it.

"What?" I ask. But Anne has already shoved her phone back into her jacket pocket.

"She was angry about the flash?"

"Since when does Anne need a reason to be angry? She told me later that Dad knew the photo album they were putting together was for his funeral. And that my snapping pics like that was disrespectful to him."

"The album was ... for his funeral?"

"I guess they were sitting around, with him right there, agreeing on what photos they would use for the funeral."

"Before he even died?"

"That's what she said."

"Wait. What?"

"My exact, same reaction, Doc."

The more I think about it, Anne's eruption over my talk with JoAnna was probably building up for a long time. Maybe from as far back as when she and I were kids. Or even further. Like those old photos in the box. Forced, frozen smiles covering up the same story. Dad was an alcoholic. His dad was an alcoholic. His grandfather was an alcoholic. They all had heart attacks, too, right around the same age, all of them mean fucking bastards with nice wives. Even Mom's dad. To hear the Aunts tell it: Grandma was nice. Grandpa always yelled. But you had to understand, he had it rough. Just like *his* father had it rough.

So that excuses everything, see?

We're at Sue's again. It's the next morning. JoAnna and I sit at the table, drinking coffee, talking about deafness and the things I haven't told her about yet. Like airports. Tell the desk clerk you're deaf, and they'll assume you need a wheelchair. It's not that Hearing people are stupid, they know the difference between deafness and paralysis. But changing policies costs money. You have to remember, though: It's your choice, whether you sit in that chair or not.

We talk about unemployment rates in the Deaf Community, underemployment rates. Suicide rates. "But thank God you graduated from high school before all of this hit," I tell her. "Because mainstreaming sucks and kids are psychotic. The bullying in mainstream schools is ..."

Of course Anne is suddenly there, out of nowhere, stomping down the stairs, stomping across the room, stomping in between us to shut this conversation down.

She is Anne.

"JoAnna," she signs, speaking simultaneously, slowly and clearly, making sure we all have full, uncontested access to her viewpoint, "Dan is angry. Dan had a hard life. The simple truth is that four out of five Hearing people are going to love you and want to help you and want to work with you. Dan lives his life focusing on that one Hearing person in five. Everything he does, everything he says and feels, is structured around that one person. But you don't have to do that, JoAnna. You have a choice. *You* can choose to be *happy*."

"My God."
"Oh, it gets much worse."

JoAnna and I are both too stunned to speak. My cheeks sting and go numb. Anne stomps away into the living room, irritated that I've made her do this, pushed it this far, brought it to this point.

The poor thing. She's had it so *hard*.

"Excuse me?" I shout at her. She snaps around, exasperated. But afraid, too. I can feel it. *"What did you just say?"*

Anne doesn't answer.

JoAnna is right there. So I hold back from saying more.

"I'm sorry, Dan. Oh my Goodness."

"I thought at first she set it up that way. You know? Picked her worst shit to say right then, in front of JoAnna, so I'd be stuck. And look weak."

"But that's not so?"

"We had to leave a few minutes later for the nursing home. It was our last day in Wisconsin. Both of us were flying out that night."

"I don't follow."

"We both drove to the nursing home together in the same car. Just the two of us. She knew we'd be alone."

I grab the wheel once we get out of town. Nothing but corn around us. Anne yells at me to *let the fuck go! Let go!* But I won't. She has to stop. I don't care if we go in the ditch.

"Motherfucker," I snarl at her. "What the fuck is your problem?"

"Let go of the wheel!"

I lean over and yank the keys from the ignition. "Either you or I are walking. Decide. Or you are telling me straight up, right now. What is going on in your fucked up head?"

"You and your shit are what's wrong!"

"My shit?"

"JoAnna needs hope! She's just a baby! You can't dump your doom and gloom on her like this!"

"She's twenty-five years old, Anne! She wants to know. She asked me to tell her!"

"She's overwhelmed! She just lost her hearing! Think about her feelings!"

"The world isn't going away! It is what it is regardless of how she feels!"

"It's not about *you*! Or that mountain-sized chip on your shoulder, you bitter, selfish prick! Or Scott! Life is different now! People know more about deafness than Mom and Dad did! She won't go through the same things!"

"She's already going through the same things!"

"How?"

"Goddamn! It's amazing, the way you are."

"What! What am I? Let's have it!"

"Your denial!"

"*My* denial?"

"If JoAnna was gay," I say, "And she had come to you. And the two of you were sitting there, instead. Talking about the difficulties of coming out to your parents as a young gay person. And suicide rates among gay teens. Or discrimination on the job. Whatever!"

"What does that have to do with anything?"

"Imagine you're talking. And Scott, staunch fucking Republican. Conservative values. About as homophobic as it gets out here in Redneck, Wisconsin! Imagine he barged into your private conversation and said '*Anne is maaad!*' And that four out of five straight people are gonna love JoAnna and want to help her! You really think that's true?"

"One's got nothing to do with the other! I don't know what the fuck you're talking about!"

I throw the keys at her.

She won't look at me.

Useless.

"*Maybe it wasn't, though.*"

"*She's a brick wall, Doc.*"

Everyone shows up at the nursing home eventually. Mom, the Aunts, the Cousins. There's a big birthday-looking cake for Dad, which I think is stupid—*Congratulations on living!*—but whatever. I keep my mouth shut, and watch more football. Then reruns of football on the news.

Good doggy.

But the clock keeps ticking. My flight out is at 5:30. David and Sue will drive us both. It'll take an hour to get to Milwaukee, another to get through security. We have to leave by three.

I can't put it off anymore.

All around us, Hearing people yapping, yapping. Scooping up Death Cake.

I find Anne. "*Hey,*" I sign. "*We need to get rid of everyone.*"

She flares up, and signs back: "*I don't need to do anything.*"

I breathe in slowly, tiny sips of breath. *Even now. Even now.* She's being like this. "Anne." I sign. "We have to leave for the airport. I am going to say goodbye to Dad, with or without you. I am not going to have the entire extended family staring at me while I do this. I want you to stand outside of the room and wait until I call for you to come in. I will say what I have to say. Then you listen to him and tell me what he says."

Prior to that moment, I don't think Anne ever truly hated me. But now? I have no doubt.

"Or you can leave him unable to tell me," I sign. "Your choice. I don't give a fuck."

I give her three seconds. Then turn to address the room. But she steps forward before I can, and speaks to them. Nicely, respectfully. People begin to clear out.

When they're gone, she stands outside the door to his room. Gestures that she's ready.

I tell him what I have to say. Nobody but me will ever know what that is.

His blue gray lips move. I motion for Anne to come in. She leans down, listens to him.

"*He says he's sorry,*" she signs. "*He says 'I love you.'*"

So that's that. Fair enough. More than I expected.

I back away, out of the room. Sue is crying. Scott stands stoically behind her.

I walk down the hall. To be alone. I was always so afraid of Anne, growing up. Now I'm afraid for her. If she pushes me again, I'm afraid of what I'll do.

"*Did she ever push you again?*"

"*Of course she did. But that was over text. She was back in California by then. I stopped responding and blocked her. Been ten years now.*"

"*I'm sorry.*"

"*It's not much different, to be honest. We never talked much before, either. Except there's no game around it now, no accident. It's intentional. She reached out once. When Mom was dying. Said we had to resolve things for Mom's sake.*"

"*You had no interest in reconciliation?*"

"*We couldn't get an interpreter for Mom's funeral. Just like at Dad's.*"

Small town bullshit, you know? Lack of resources. Anne texted Marie. Offered to sign at the service, since Marie couldn't go. I took Marie's phone and texted back. Told her it was me replying. Said that if she signed at the funeral, I couldn't stop her, but I wouldn't look, and wouldn't talk to her. So just stay away."

"When did your mother pass?"

"Three years back."

"A long time."

"Anne will survive."

"Still."

"Anne doesn't need anyone."

"People need other people, Dan."

"Dogs aren't people."

"You aren't a dog."

"Exactly."

The Kitchen Helper

Mamma told me to go make a bowl of salad for the table.
Mamma told me again to go set the table.
Mamma told me to bring the food to the table.
Now that everyone sat ready around the table,
They started eating and talking straightaway.
I asked what's the topic about?
They told me that it's nothing important for me to know.
I was just a server to them.

My Dearest Friend

While my family conversed on many different topics,
Gossiping about people and their family business,
I went to meet my dear friend in the other room
Where I missed out on their boring talk.

Ah. Finally I was able to meet my dear friend.
No, actually my dearest friend, who kept me sane,
Who entertained me,
Who showed me fascinating things,
Who showed me how people socialized,
Who educated me on nature, animals, everything,
Who gave me comedy so I could laugh out loud.
I had no one else to hang out with me.
My dearest friend's name was
T-E-L-E-V-I-S-I-O-N.

Carnaval, Upstate

I ran home from the bus stop, the cold mineral air of winter filling my lungs. Laughter vibrated in my throat as I passed our neighbor's powder-blue house with Christmas lights sagging over their front windows. I almost slipped on a patch of slush before catching myself. I didn't care that it was February in Syracuse, the worst month of all with its dirty brown snow and dirty gray skies. None of that mattered because today was Carnaval.

Panting, I stopped outside of the screen door to what used to be my only home. There was so much to tell Mamãe and Papai. About the swimming pool and the library at my new residential school. About how Shannon was my best friend now. About how there was a Deaf world and how different it was. But not about Kyle or what I had said to Shannon. These I would keep to myself.

I opened the door, and warmth covered my face as Mamãe smiled up at me. Her mouth shaped some words that escaped me. Before I could figure them out, she swept me into her arms.

I must've gotten worse at lip-reading. I kept thinking about what she said, like playing a videotape over and over in my head. Then I think I got it: "You're finally home! Tell us everything."

Papai's glasses bumped my head as he hugged us. I breathed in his smell of laundry detergent as their arms encircled me. I was home now. Papai looked the same with his big dorky glasses and the blue button-down shirts he bought in bulk from K-Mart. His chest rumbled like he was talking. Sometimes he forgot that I couldn't hear him.

I told them how much I missed them and how wonderful yet strange school was. They stared at me in that confused way they had when someone spoke English too fast. It's funny how much you forget when you go away. Here, I used English or my voice. ASL was for school. I arranged signs in a more English way, which felt slow and clumsy. That didn't work either, so I spoke, twisting my tongue and trying to breathe right. The words finally came, "I missed you." I forgot how hard using my voice was.

They understood and hugged me again.

I inhaled to say more, but Papai walked away before I could stop him. When he picked up the phone, I understood. I wished they would tell me about things like when the phone rings. Anger bubbled up in me. This never happened at school.

It took a while for Mamãe to fingerspell *Roberto*, her fingers tripping over one another. She wasn't practicing, which meant she would forget everything. I was about to scold her until I saw the dried blood around her nails. She was working extra hours, washing dishes and scrubbing floors—for Papai and me. It wasn't a good time to talk.

I wanted to tell her what it was like at my new school, Rochester School of the Deaf, where I started eighth grade this year. Everyone used my sign name, *M* at the corner of the mouth, instead of just calling me Marina like hearing people do. Everyone talked so much there, words flowing so fast that it made me dizzy. Sometimes I didn't know what to say, like with Kyle and Shannon, which is strange since I'm supposed to know how to talk to everyone there.

RSD was nothing like my old school where everyone was hearing, which was all right for a while. Some kids learned signs like "turtle" and "poop," good enough for us to talk a little and play games like Spit. That changed last year, though. My best friend Delia started saying that it was rude to point and make faces, but that's how sign language works. The other girls only talked about boys, usually forgetting to face me so I could lip-read, and kept laughing without telling me why.

I told Alice about this when she came for our weekly meetings. She was my teacher of the deaf who knew about Deaf things, and the school administration said she would help me achieve my full potential—whatever that meant. After I talked about how Delia had hurt my feelings, Alice looked sad. "She's hearing," she said. "It's hard for hearing people to understand what it's like having to try so hard to communicate." That was when she told me about RSD.

When I asked to go there, Mamãe cried, and Papai said that the education wasn't good. I told them that I wanted to be somewhere everyone understood each other. I don't know if that's what happened.

Carnaval was in the air. *Feijoada* bubbled on the stove, filling the basement with the smell of beans, onions, and meat. Bright reds and blues covered up the awful beige walls our landlord wouldn't let us paint. Carnaval was better than Christmases and birthdays because you celebrated surrounded by dancing. When I described this to Shannon, she said that the costumes sounded weird. Kyle laughed at the idea of clowns at my house, even though I had explained that it wasn't like American carnivals.

Carnaval means happiness and new beginnings. You dance when it's cold and gray outside. Everyone dresses up to welcome the spring together. Maybe it's different in Brazil since it's summer there when it's winter here.

Mamãe snatched a feather from Papai with that mad-annoyed look that she got when I forgot to take out the trash. Their mouths moved in that Portuguese way. Papai touched her cheek and said something that made her stop waving the feather. She didn't look happy, but she didn't look mad either. I wished I knew what he had said. I forgot most of my Portuguese after I got sick and went deaf when I was two. Teachers told my parents that they should only speak English with me. Something about how English and sign language were more important. So that's why they use only English with me even though they're lousy at it. Sometimes Mamãe speaks Portuguese by accident and cries when she realizes her mistake.

As she hung paper palm trees, Mamãe's hips swung like a pendulum, gentle and soothing. Papai bobbed his head in that dorky way of his. I was thinking about how silly they looked when I understood. Music was playing, too quiet for me to feel.

Before I could ask them to turn up the music, Mamãe's mouth outlined something like *dress* before sashaying down the hallway. Papai crouched by the big stereo, wires dangling from his mouth with a crumpled manual next to him. Even though he's good at science, Papai's no good with machines. He broke the furnace once, and we had to sleep in our parkas for a week. He seemed too busy to talk, so I followed Mamãe.

She sat behind a pastel-green sewing machine with pins sticking out from her mouth. She looked so peaceful that I didn't want to spoil it. She was making one of her creations, clothes that belonged in fancy stores with shiny floors.

She could be more than a housekeeper. I once found a photograph of her standing next to a tall blonde wearing a yellow dress that floated around her body like a cloud of daisies. It said, "Rio Fashion Week 1984" at the bottom, which was the year before I was born. When I asked her why she didn't go to New York to show her dresses, she looked sad and fingerspelled "Can't. Love you both too much." Now she babysits and cleans "under the table" because Papai is here on a student visa.

She slid the fabric into the machine, her fingers so close to the needle that it looked like she'd hurt herself, but she didn't. Every stitch was perfect. A soft smile grew on her face that made her look younger and not so tired. When she looked up and saw me, the smile changed. I can't explain how, just that it did.

She snipped a thread, and the dress was done. She wriggled into it, and I gasped. It was one of her best. Reds and purples swirled around her hips and breasts, making her look curvier and taller. After I fastened the back, she twirled and her mouth moved, "You like?"

My fingers swept around my face: *beautiful.*

Her eyes lit up, and the soft smile returned. She remembered the sign.

She pointed at the mirror, and her lips moved, "Same. We the same."

We looked more alike than I remembered with our thick black hair and lips that pouted without looking sad. Up close, I saw how different we were. Her lips bright with lipstick and eyelashes heavy with mascara, she was so dazzling that I almost didn't notice the wrinkles around her eyes. I looked plain with my face bare of color and jeans that sagged at the knees. She wore a gorgeous painting.

"I want to dance in a dress like yours," I said, the words thick in my mouth.

Her hand went to my cheek. "Later. Too young."

I scowled at my reflection. I hadn't been too young to have a boy slide a hand up my shirt last week.

When Kyle led me to an empty room after class, I thought he wanted to ask me about an essay on *Shiloh*. Instead, he asked if he could kiss me. After thinking about it, I said yes. I wanted to know what it was like.

It felt like an alien ship landing on my mouth that tasted like warm orange juice. I didn't like it at first, then I understood why all of the girls talked about kissing. It was like the heat from his mouth spread throughout my body, warming up all of me. That felt good, so good that I wanted more. So I let him lift up my shirt and put his mouth on my breasts.

The next morning, the other boys waggled their eyebrows as I walked by. The girls turned away, but I saw their hands twisting at their cheeks: *slut*. I never told anyone about the kiss, so Kyle must have.

Kyle isn't popular just because he plays basketball and looks like Leonardo DiCaprio, except with dark eyes and hair that's always in his eyes. He comes from a Deaf family, which means that his parents, grandparents, and even great-grandparents are all Deaf. His parents are important people. His dad teaches at the university, and his mom does what they call advocacy work. Shannon said that this is the best kind of family because everyone understands each other.

I found Mamãe and Papai in the living room, arms wrapped around each other as they danced. The only time that Papai danced well was with Mamãe. Otherwise, he bobbed his head like a duck. She said that it was because he was from São Paulo. "They too serious. We Rio people know how to have fun!" They must've forgotten I was there because they looked like they would kiss, so I left. It never seemed like the right time to talk to them.

Half of the living room was now in my bedroom. A couch leaned against the wall, surrounded by boxes full of Papai's textbooks. Mamãe's mannequins blocked the way to my bed. I missed my bed at school where Shannon and I talked after lights out using a flashlight.

When I first arrived at school, Shannon grabbed my hand and showed me around. Even though she looks like a popular girl with the way she walks with her back straight and head thrown back, she's not stuck-up. She showed me the classrooms, told me which teachers would let you hand in homework late like Mr. Titus and who wouldn't like Ms. Rausch, and to say "I'm Deaf, too" if I saw another Deaf person. We talked about who was cute, like Kyle, and who wasn't, like Barry. When she invited me to her home three weeks ago, I said yes.

She lived in a big house in Buffalo with four bedrooms, a silvery kitchen, and a finished basement with a big TV. Shannon's mom was really pretty in that magazine kind of way where she wore clothes with boring colors like gray or taupe but somehow looked beautiful. When she brought us hot chocolate, she moved her mouth in that careful way people use with Deaf people, which made Shannon embarrassed for some reason. Her mom was good at it though, and didn't speak too slowly or make weird faces. That's why I understood her at dinner.

Shannon was slouching at the dinner table when her mom said, "Shannon, have you been practicing?" with a teacher-type of look. "It's important to keep up your articulation." Shannon's face reddened and she yelled, "I told you! No more!" with her hands flying. She ran off and slammed the door so hard the floor shook.

Her mom turned to me with that confused expression that you see on foreigners, which looked all wrong on her face. I think she wanted to ask what Shannon said because her fingers twitched like she wanted to sign but she picked up the dirty plates instead. Before she walked away, I saw tears in her eyes.

I had never seen Shannon so upset before. Her hand almost hit the lamp as she told me about the speech lessons. "My mom says I'm not trying hard enough. I tried so hard! I'm just not good at it." She opened and closed her mouth in a way that made speaking look ridiculous and paused like she was thinking hard. "She's not really my family. You and I are a real family. We understand each other."

Her hands drew a circle in the air between us, like we belonged together. I thought of how much I liked talking to her and the other kids at school. They didn't say things like "Never mind," or "It's not important." My hands could move as fast as my thoughts, and their eyes never got that confused look. I hugged Shannon and told her we were a family.

When we went to sleep, I thought of Mamãe and Papai, their eyes full of hurt. If I were part of the Deaf family, how could I still be part of theirs? I lay awake, wondering how to fit two circles together.

Now, Shannon was mad at me. When I said that I wanted to tell off Kyle for blabbing, she shook her head. "You have a chance to get the perfect family, so don't screw it up!" she said. She didn't hug me goodbye before I left, and I didn't know what to say to either one of them.

I was flipping through one of Papai's textbooks about something called quantum mechanics when I felt the vibrations—the bed shaking to the beat of samba drums. Carnaval was finally here! I flung open the door, and the vibrations hit me in the chest. People had their hands in the air, swaying to the music that pounded throughout my body. Roberto waved at me from the corner, a big smile on his face.

I've always thought Roberto was good-looking, maybe even better looking than Kyle. He's skinny with curly black hair tied back in a ponytail, which doesn't make him look like a girl at all. He smiles at you like he wants to be your friend. Kyle smiles like he has lots of friends already.

"You're back! How's school?" he signed.

I pressed my cheek against his chest and inhaled his smell—Pert shampoo mixed with something spicy. I forgot for a moment that I had been away.

Roberto had moved in upstairs when he was a graduate student and never left, even though he's a teacher now. He watched me whenever my parents had to work, which was a lot. He learned to talk with me, and now he can sign really well for a hearing person. He said it was because he plays guitar. I think it's something else.

"School's good," I said, trying not to think about the boys' waggling eyebrows.

"You're so far away. It's too quiet here now."

I thought about telling him everything. About how the other kids asked me if my family sold drugs. About what happened with Shannon. About how everyone had changed my sign name to *slut*. About how I felt different from the other kids even though we're all Deaf. But I couldn't.

When I was little, I imagined Roberto and me living upstairs, and my parents living downstairs. We would have Carnaval parties every year with him translating for all of us. It would be perfect, and if I told him, it would ruin everything. I didn't know why, just that it would.

"Are you enjoying the party?" I asked instead.

A dimple appeared in his left cheek. "It reminds me of the discotheques in Mexico City." He gyrated like John Travolta, making me giggle.

His eyes got serious. His hands moved—"Tell me more about school"—until he caught sight of a blonde wearing a skirt too short for Syracuse winters. He promised to talk later and went to the blonde. She kept flipping her hair, which made her look like she had a neck problem. Roberto must've liked it, though, since they went upstairs together. Maybe she was his girlfriend, and he hadn't told me.

Bodies and colors swirled around me as people talked, laughed, and danced. Lips shaped into different languages. Portuguese had more lip-puckering and moved faster. English was slower, with the mouth opening wider. Spanish was somewhere in between. No matter how hard I tried, the words stayed out of my reach.

I bumped against a table full of *caipirinhas*. Papai likes to drink them and say, "Only real Brazilians drink these. Americans keep their watery beers and snobby wines." His eyes always glazed over, and he acted like he didn't have to worry about money or his dissertation.

I stared into the cup, wondering what it tasted like. Everyone said that drinking was bad. Teachers. Roberto. Mamãe and Papai. The word *no* appeared in my mind, the oval mouth-shape, the fingers clamping together. I wanted to tell everyone *no*. No to Mamãe and Papai for not understanding me. No to Kyle for blabbing. No to the name-calling at school. No to Roberto for not telling me about his girlfriend. No, no, no!

The drink burned all the way down. How could Papai like something so awful? I must've missed something, so I drank another and another. It was like kissing. The more I tried it, the more I liked it. The sweet and tart blended into something so delicious that nothing else mattered.

Nobody noticed. Everyone kept dancing, dancing, dancing.

The floor turned wobbly like jelly. A red feather bounced in the air, so beautiful, and a pleasant heaviness weighed down my limbs. Somehow the colors, the movements, everything around me, had become more vivid, more *real*.

BOOM, badum—badum—tish. BOOM, badum—badum—tish.

The beat flowed through my body, the drums pounding as I swayed, swayed. Everyone was twisting and turning, the colors of their masks blurring together. It felt like we were living inside one of Mamãe's dresses with colors floating all around us.

BOOM, badum—badum—tish. BOOM, badum—badum—tish.

Expressions of ecstasy surrounded me as everyone lost themselves in the dance. Oh, I wanted to reach out and touch their happiness, or maybe I could. I didn't just want to watch, not anymore.

Cuica—cuica—BRRRUUUU—UUM! BOOM, badum—badum—tish. BOOM, badum—badum—tish.

I wanted to dance. Why hadn't I thought of this before? It was so obvious! The drums inside me had to escape, I needed to go out there and dance, dance, dance.

Hot, sweaty bodies pressed against me. I raised my arms and waited for the dance to come. Nothing happened ... my body wouldn't move ... a man looked angry when I stepped on his foot ... I'm sorry ... I tried to follow everyone else ... I tried harder ... stiff limbs ... nothing was working!

Tears stung the back of my eyes. I turned and saw her.

Mamãe was dancing on top of a table, her hips whirling in figure-eights. The lines of her dress swirled together into whirlpools of color. Oh! So beautiful. A smile lifted her mouth as she reached up. Oh! The picture was interrupted when Papai brought her down to dance with him. They swayed together in perfect harmony.

The table stood empty, looking sad. Mouths opened in "Dance! Dance!" I took an outstretched hand and jumped onto the table. Everything started to spin, and I squeezed my eyes shut. The music felt shaper, clearer here. *Cuica—cuica—BRRRUUUU.* My body loosened, moving to the beat pulsing upward. *Badum—badum—BOOM.* Yes, yes, yes! Sway, lift, shimmy, twirl. I was dancing! Dancing, dancing, dancing!

Rum—brum—BRRRRUUUUU—UUM!

Laughter burst out of me. The dance flowed through me, bringing with it everyone's joy. I belonged here. Twirling, twirling, twirling.

Something grabbed me and I almost fell off the table.

Papai's hand was on my arm—why?—and he swept me off the table. His hand kept me in place as Mamãe's worried face appeared. Her lips moved in meaningless shapes, nonsense, gibberish. I shook my head. What did she say? What was happening?

Hands—theirs? someone else's?—pushed and pulled at me. Papai's glasses flashed the reflection of Carnaval's colors. Everything went double, two of Papai and Mamãe, four anxious faces, six mouths flapping in nonsensical shapes. What? Why? The harder I tried to catch the words, the more they slipped away. I was sick of always chasing the mouth-shapes, trying so hard to understand, of not being understood. Enough!

My fingers moved—flying, swooping, dancing—as my words flowed in torrents. Why don't you know my language? Don't you know what that means? It means that you don't know the Deaf world, you can't understand me, and if you don't understand who I am, how can you love me? How can we be a real family? My hands danced in the air, all of my thoughts unleashed, free of slow movements and cramped tongues. Don't you understand, Mamãe and Papai? Don't you want to be my family?

Someone jostled me, breaking the circle I was drawing in the air. Papai looked like someone had punched him. Mamãe put her face into her hands, her shoulders shaking like she was crying. They stayed there, looking small and broken. Even if they didn't understand the words, they felt their force.

Everyone kept dancing around us, making me dizzy and queasy. My stomach cramped as I circled my fist on my chest—I'm sorry—and ran, ran to the bathroom. I was going to be sick.

The white bottom of the toilet bowl gleamed as Mamãe held my hair back. My stomach clenched and everything came up. My mouth burned afterward. Papai's arm felt warm around my shoulder as I fell into their bed.

I woke up with a dry mouth and a throbbing headache. Mamãe was sitting by me with a glass of water and an aspirin, her face scrubbed clean. She looked younger, more like me. I gulped down the water, the most refreshing thing I had ever tasted. She started to talk, her hands too slow for her mouth. I was too young to drink. Carnaval wasn't an excuse to misbehave. I had to clean up the mess as punishment. That was what she said, more or less.

She pressed her cool hand to my forehead, her eyes full of melancholy as if she wished for something she could never have. Her lips moved in that Portuguese way and I caught a word, amor, love. The strange expression vanished, and her palms came together, "Clean up now!"

My head pounded as I went into the living room. It was a mess. Empty paper plates and cups were everywhere, even on the new stereo, which had a big brown puddle on top. I hoped Papai hadn't seen that yet. My foot caught onto some lumps in the carpet. Someone had stepped on some pão de queijo and smashed it deep into the fibers.

I felt footsteps behind me and turned to see Roberto. "Crazy Carnaval this year, uh?" he said after hugging me. "Sorry that I missed your dance show."

My blush made him laugh.

"We all need a release sometimes. Otherwise, you're too bottled up to think straight. Things look better afterward," he said before grabbing an overflowing trash bag and heading outside.

Papai came to kiss my forehead. His eyes had the same sadness as Mamãe's had. Maybe they understood what I had told them yesterday—not everything, but enough. And they still loved me.

The vacuum rumbled as I passed it over shreds of feathers and fallen confetti. As I cleaned, my thoughts untangled, and I finally knew what to say. To Kyle, I would say that it doesn't matter that he's popular because I don't kiss blabbermouths. To Shannon, I would explain that I don't need perfect families, just a real friend. That made me feel better, ready to go back.

I turned off the vacuum when it reached two paper plates on the carpet, stacked like a Venn diagram. I picked them up and tried to mash them together, but they crumpled without merging. I stared down at the crushed circles that would never become one and put one on top of the other. Maybe this was just how things were. Two circles, two families, and two lives. Two was more than one, and maybe that wasn't so bad.

JER LOUDENBACK

Family Language

At age 7,
I was deprived of my true language.
The family dinner table stood
right at my nose.
My plate had a fork on the left,
a spoon and knife on the right.
A napkin sat on the right.
I gazed up at my family
as they spoke.
Their mouths moved beautifully.
Even though I didn't understand,
I still gazed in wonder.

At age 12,
I was not so deprived of my true language.
It had begun to grow inside me.
I had grown tall enough
to sit and look across the 3-D landscape
of plates, forks, spoons, and knives.
I could now see shadows underneath
the plates and silverware:
more depth.
I watched my family,
their mouths still moving like before.
Could I lipread and understand?
Not if they spoke so fast.
Always a curious person,
I asked what they were talking about.
They used gestures to communicate with me.
They always held up an index finger.
That meant, *Wait*.
Again: *Wait*.
Again: Wait.
I thought their finger pointing up was a sign of God

coming down to push me down
into silence.

At age 18,
I had grown more into my true language.
I had become more aware of my environment
and its many languages.
Having decorated the holiday table,
my family seemed more animated.
I saw more colors all over.
My family still spoke, their mouths moving.
They never stopped.
Still a curious person, I asked many questions.
Their answers remained the same:
Their fingers said, *Wait.*
Then they said, "I'll tell you later."
Did I get the answers I needed
for my intellect to grow and thrive?
No.
I didn't feel just deflated,
but even more deflated to the core of my soul.

At age 25,
I had already graduated from college.
One day my hearing family called me on my TTY.
They wanted to invite me over for dinner.
At that moment I thought back to the many years
I'd sat with them and suffered
from not understanding them
and feeling deflated over and over again.
I typed, If I do come over, will you share
all the conversations you've had
since I was little and missed out on?
Can you, or will you?
They did not respond.
I hung up on my TTY.

After so many years,
I finally felt freed of my suffering.
Yet all the family connections
I had wanted faded away.
My language of freedom had turned powerful.

Lucky

The lights flickering on and off broke through my sleep. I looked at the clock on the table next to my bed. Just after 6:00. I rolled over and pulled the covers over my head. Through them and my closed eyes, I could still see the light go on and stay on. I felt the vibrations of someone walking into my room. The person poked me on the shoulder.

"I'm tired. Let me sleep," I said without looking to see who had woken me up. If I just kept my eyes closed, I didn't need to engage.

But then whoever it was yanked the covers off, so I sat up and opened my eyes. My brother Henry stood next to my bed still holding my green-and-white checked comforter in his hands. "Mom says to come to dinner."

"Tell her I'm too tired. I'm not hungry." I grabbed the bedclothes back and resettled myself. Henry walked out but left the lights on and my door open. I pulled the covers over my head and turned on my side away from the door, hiding my head in my arms to block the light. That worked OK, but nothing could block the inviting smells coming from the kitchen: the garlic, tomato, and hamburger that meant Mom's spaghetti meat sauce, the toasted garlic bread, even the cooked-pasta smell.

Tempting! But I really was tired. Dealing with hearing people all day at school took a lot of energy. The lipreading was part of it. So was the constant need to be alert to environmental cues around me. And on top of that, the simple emotional drain of being different from everyone else in such an obvious way. Dinner with my family—Mom, two brothers, and two sisters—required the same kinds of work. I needed the break from working hard to understand my hearing family and the frustration and feelings of isolation when inevitably I didn't understand. Mom also had a predictably unpredictable temper; the best way to avoid getting yelled at, threatened, and punished was to avoid being in the same room.

Someone sat down on my bed, put a hand on my shoulder, and gently shook it. Mom—which I knew even before I rolled onto my back so I could see her.

"Henry said you don't want to come to dinner."

"I'm too tired."

"But then you miss out on family time."

That's the goal, I thought, but wisely said nothing.

"You're not setting a good example for your sisters."

But a good example for Henry and Todd? Even my sarcastic brain knew the explanation: My brothers were only 14 months and two-and-a-half years younger than me, while my sisters were six-and-a-half and nine years younger. I did a lot of unpaid babysitting!

"You have to stop doing this. If you have so much to do that you're too tired for family time, you can't go over to Kathy's on Saturday."

I gambled that Mom would forget about not letting me go over to my best friend's house. "I'm too tired," I repeated and rolled back onto my side.

Mom did her annoying thing of making little cross motions on my ear that she could reach, like a priest putting ashes on foreheads on Ash Wednesday. She believed God would heal me, make me hear again.

Later, after dinner was long cleared, I got up to get something to eat. I didn't see any leftovers in the fridge, so I made myself a sandwich. I got my book of the moment, *A Confederacy of Dunces.* Kathy's English teacher assigned it, and she didn't like it. My teacher didn't assign it, but I borrowed her copy at school during lunch and read the first few pages. I had to read it! I stopped at The Little Professor bookstore down the street from our high school on the way home to buy it. The store had an agreement with the school to stock the books our teacher wanted to teach that the New Orleans Public Schools didn't stock as textbooks. I ate and laughed at the antics of Ignatius J. Reilly.

Books never got mad at me or made me wait for later to know what was going on or laughed so hard they couldn't tell me what the joke was. And I didn't have to work hard to figure out what they said. Although I hated for good books to end, I could always re-read a book if I didn't want to lose its companionship. Dinner with the family wouldn't have been too bad if Mom had let me read a book at the table, but she said it was rude.

My nap-while-doing-homework strategy didn't work on weekends. I didn't seem to need it as much at Dad's house. Even in retrospect, I'm not sure why. Part is likely that I didn't have to walk on eggshells with Dad, so I was only dealing with communication barriers, not communication barriers plus fearing that I might inadvertently bring down parental wrath. But it might also be that there were so many of us at my Dad's table—Dad, his five kids, my stepmother, and her two kids—that there was no single conversation to follow. I could get into a conversation I could manage with just one or two of the other people at the table. No one was "in" all of the conversations.

But at Mom's, I'd be balancing spending energy to be included while also not saying or doing the wrong thing to set Mom off. I mean, I remember one time at dinner I mentioned what I'd been reading for my English class, Swift's "A Modest Proposal," because I was impressed with it. Good satire is hard to pull off! I explained that it is a satirical proposal that the Irish should fatten up their babies and sell them to the English as a delicacy. They'd reduce the mouths to feed and also make a profit! This was for the benefit of my siblings—since they were behind me in school, they hadn't arrived at Swift yet. I just assumed Mom would have read it, too! But Mom blew up at me for talking about something so awful.

One Saturday, dinner was later than usual; we didn't sit down for dinner until it was almost time for Mom's radio show, *A Prairie Home Companion*. I was vaguely aware that Mom listened to this show every week. It seemed to make her feel connected to her Illinois farm upbringing, the same nostalgia for "country" that was evident in her collection of chickens and roosters (even though her family hadn't raised chickens). But usually, it was something Mom listened to after dinner when I'd be on kitchen cleanup (a chore my siblings and I rotated—one to clear the table, one to wash dishes, one to dry and put them away) or with my nose in a book. Sometimes I watched TV with my siblings if there was something on that I wanted to watch that was captioned and also met Mom's approval. There were more choices now that Mom had finally gotten cable so that she could watch her TV preachers.

After she said grace, Mom got up and walked into the kitchen, which was separated from the dining room by a counter. She went over to the refrigerator, but instead of getting food, she reached up to the radio on the top. I assumed it had been on and she was turning it off. She had so many times made it clear she looked down on all the families that have televisions in their eating areas and watch TV while they eat instead of talking to each other. (See "Ban on reading at the table.")

I didn't see anyone talking at the table, so I decided to start a conversation. One thing about lipreading is that it is much easier if you control (or at least know) the topic. This was in the fall of 1984, and I was excited there was finally a woman on a major party ticket. It was also my semester for taking the required Civics class in high school, and I was working on a project to make campaign posters. Maybe in some families, politics would be the wrong topic, but for us (for my mom!) it seemed safe. She initially supported Jesse Jackson and his Rainbow Coalition (giving him one of the votes that gave him the Louisiana primary win) but she'd be voting for the Mondale-Ferraro ticket come November. The polls didn't give them a real chance, but maybe the next election, when I'd actually be able to vote, we'd get our first female VP—or even President. Why not? Great Britain had Margaret Thatcher.

"Mom," I started.

Mom held up a finger to her lips. "Shhhh. We're listening to the radio."

"You're listening to the radio?" I didn't really question if I had lipread Mom correctly. What I really wondered was how she could think it was a good idea to ask her deaf daughter to just sit there while the radio entertained everyone else at the table.

"Yes, shhh." Mom repeated the gesture to be quiet.

I wish I could say that I called Mom on the utter unfairness of expecting me to be quiet so she could listen to the radio, but I just sat there. Anger killed my appetite, but I put food in my mouth, chewed, and swallowed just for something to do and to keep myself from crying. Every seat at our table was full, but I was alone.

Looking back, I probably wouldn't have enjoyed the radio show much. When I was twenty, someone gave me a copy of Garrison Keillor's *Lake Wobegon Days*, so I read it. I could see why Mom enjoyed his radio shows, but Keillor wasn't my thing. My siblings probably weren't thrilled with having to listen to Mom's show while they ate. Maybe they were envious of me not having to listen. I certainly had the advantage for tuning Mom out. Same battlefield, different experiences because of position. Lucky me!

After I left home and joined the Deaf community, I realized that for a nonsigning hearing family, my siblings were actually pretty good about making sure I knew what was going on. Usually, I didn't need to ask them to fill me in, at least not with words. I'd tilt my head to the side and raise my eyebrows, and one of them would fill me in. They had plenty of practice since we ate all meals together when we were home—so pretty much always dinner, and breakfast and lunch too on weekends and holidays. (This was pretty much the same at Dad's house, but after my parents split up he had us only every other weekend, so we had much less time with him.)

I missed my siblings when I left for college, but I didn't miss the mix of dealing with being deaf in a hearing family in a household led by someone who wanted family togetherness her way. After I left for college, I only came home for some holidays, and only for one summer. When I came home for Christmas in my senior year, it had been a full year since I'd been home.

By the time my family sat down to Christmas dinner that year, all my siblings and I wanted to do was eat and get the kitchen cleaned up so we could open our gifts. It was already midafternoon and many hours past the traditional Christmas cinnamon roll breakfast before Christmas Mass. We had had hours of smelling the turkey roasting.

We couldn't just start heaping food onto our fancy china plates, though. Every meal at our house started with grace. I looked toward Mom at my left, at the head of the table, for the ending "in the name of the Father, the Son, and the Holy Spirit. Amen" and its helpful accompanying crossing gesture (which we all did, more or less in sync).

I reached out for the serving dish closest to me but Mom reached out to stop me.

I looked at her lips. I'm an unusually good lipreader, and especially good at understanding Mom when I tried and when she wasn't covering her mouth. "Before we eat, I want each of us to sing a Christmas carol."

Mom went first. I didn't bother trying to read her lips while she sang. I sat there trying to think what I would do when it was my turn. If we went around the table, I'd be either next or last. I have a good-for-a-deaf-person voice, and I remember many Christmas songs from the years before I became deaf. No way would I sing for them though. It wasn't just that I couldn't tell how I sounded or that I knew I had poor volume control, but also that any time I tried to do something unusual with my voice, my throat would hurt. While Mom sang, I came to a solution. I'd sign.

"Silent Night."

Mom wrapped up with a rapturous expression. Everyone looked at me.

I started to sign: SILENT NIGHT, HOLY NIGHT.

I half-expected Mom to object, but she didn't say anything. No one else in my family signed beyond the ABCs. I had myself just really started learning when I got to college so that I could use interpreters in class. I made a Deaf friend, went to a Deaf church sometimes, and took the two semesters of ASL classes my university offered, but mostly I picked up signs from watching my interpreters. Not that it mattered here—since none of my family knew ASL, I could even do fake signs. They wouldn't know the difference.

Nevertheless, I faithfully signed "Silent Night," with an emphasis on the "silent."

When I finished, it was Emily's turn. I zoned out again and sunk into my thoughts. Did Mom really think this was the way to create happy family holiday memories? Not for the first time, I vowed to myself that if I ever had kids, we would open gifts first thing on Christmas morning, or even on Christmas Eve. I'd read that some people did that. Or they'd go to Midnight Mass and open gifts right after. The people around my table wouldn't ask me to do a hearing-people thing like sing or do so themselves oblivious of if I could understand. Not that I cared to know what Christmas carol my sister sang, but who demands a family singing activity that excludes one of the family?

My mom, apparently.

My train of thought broke when Mom's face shifted from her blissful prayer face to angry. She said something directed to Todd, who was now singing—it hadn't registered for me that Emily was done! Todd kept singing whatever he was singing. I looked back at Mom, who was now yelling something at him.

Todd stopped singing. Mom kept yelling. Henry was clearly upset. My sisters both looked ready to cry. Todd yelled back.

I wanted to know what was going on, and I didn't want to know what was going on. I had spent my last years at home counting down the time I could leave for college to escape. Four more years. Three more years. Two. One. Six months. Three months.

Mom stood up, threw the contents of her water glass at Todd, and left the room. Todd also stormed out.

"What's going on?" I asked my siblings.

"Mom wanted a religious Christmas carol. Todd sang 'Rudolf the Red-nosed Reindeer.' Mom yelled at him to stop and sing a religious one. He kept going and when he was done said she hadn't specified religious, and he wasn't going to sing another one," Henry explained.

"Mom threw a fit over that? On Christmas?" I shouldn't have been surprised, but shouldn't there be some kind of Christmas cease-fire?

"Yeah, Mom kicked Todd out. She told him to pack up his stuff and get out of the house."

"On Christmas?"

Henry went upstairs to check on Todd in the room they grew up sharing. It was now mostly Todd's since Henry had also left for the peace of college away from home. Todd was in his freshman year of college but had decided to go to the University of New Orleans and live at home to save money. My sisters said that he and Mom fought all the time.

I sat with my sisters on the sofa in our den and tried to comfort them. I was upset, too, but taking care of my little sisters was a habit. Since I also missed part of the fight and got information after the fact, that may also have softened the blow.

I hoped Mom would come out of her room, which was just off the den, and apologize to Todd and rescue our Christmas.

My brothers came downstairs. Todd carried a packed bag. He went to the phone in the kitchen, called his girlfriend to come and pick him up, and went outside to wait for her.

I went to Mom's room to check on her. I knocked on the closed door. "Mom?" I said and waited a few moments since I couldn't hear an answer. She lay in bed in her dark room. I turned on the light. Mom raised herself up a bit against the headboard, and I sat down on the edge of her bed. Her eyes were red from crying.

"Are you OK, Mom?"

She shook her head no, and a fresh tear ran down her cheek. I reached over to her bedside table for a tissue and handed it to her. She dabbed her eyes, blew her nose, and took a deep breath.

"Todd is so willful! He really hurt my feelings. Can you talk to him?"

"Mom, Todd left the house. You told him to!"

Mom didn't say anything.

"What are the rest of us supposed to do?" I asked. "It's Christmas."

"I'm sorry. I don't feel very good. I'm going to sleep. Can you make sure everyone eats?"

I nodded and got up. Mom slid back down, and I tucked the covers up around her.

"Goodnight, Mom." I turned out the light as I left the room. I closed not only her door but also the door from the den to the short hallway leading to her room and mine.

Henry, Emily, Erica, and I put up leftovers after making ourselves plates and popping them in the microwave. We ate around the small in-kitchen table—the dining room table remained set with the china. No one had much to say. I think they were as shocked as I was that Mom actually kicked one of us out after threatening that so much I had lost count.

The next morning, Todd called home to ask if he could pick up some stuff. Mom relented and told him he could come back home. We opened our Christmas gifts. By dinner, things were as usual at the table.

I couldn't wait to go back to school.

To Someone of Low Morals

I wish I could understand
what you are talking about,
when you speak of a topic
that I do not understand.

When I ask you a question
of the words you are saying,
laughter is all that I get—
as if somehow I'm stupid,
dare I even use that word.

Perhaps, the message is sent:
If I don't need to know what
you have been saying, or if
you are inappropriate
in what you are discussing,
then why should I ever ask?

Should I continue to be
associating myself
with someone of low morals?
I mean, I wouldn't want to
talk in the dirty manners
I believe you are doing.

Maybe I should consider,
although it would really hurt
to lose a friend over words
that I don't feel should be said.

The Helichloros

In outer space, Josephine Kepler knew no one could hear you scream, but when you're Deaf, it's because no one gave a damn.

She was painfully reminded of this fact once again in the *U.E.S. Athena*'s mess hall. Using a fork, she fiddled with her replicated meal. Her tower of peas overlooked her sea of smash potatoes.

Josephine watched the smiles, laughs, and questions on the faces of her colleagues trying to score scientific breakthroughs. Or at least that was her assumption since she couldn't follow their conversations. Even though the crew on *U.E.S. Athena* was quite diverse, she was the only Deaf person aboard. Not only that, her emerald eyes made her stand out because they signified her genetic lack of auditory nerves. Her lab coat hid not only her quirky, colorful overalls, but also a hologram interpreter orb which no one on the ship had cared to use.

Her brother Ethan was laughing uproariously at some joke at the table when she hesitantly nudged him. He made a face, and without missing a beat, waved her off mouthing, "Ay-uhl tel yoo lay-ter," and immediately resumed his laughing. Frowning, she nudged him again and pulled out the hologram interpreter orb from her lab coat.

Ethan Kepler, *Athena*'s Chief Science Officer, was currently sporting a puny handlebar mustache in an attempt to emulate their father's impressive painter's brush mustache. Josephine and their sister Eimy often joked about how Ethan's mustache looked drawn on with an antique permanent marker, just like the ones from vintage Earth movies that usually had no captions. Ethan wore the ship's standard white uniform with a blue vest that indicated that he belonged to the Science Department.

The orb vibrated as Ethan shook it in his hand and a human hologram projected outward. He started clicking buttons making the figure switch from Voice to Sign and back. He mumbled dismissively and threw the orb back at her. "Too hard."

She flipped him a middle finger and carried her tray to a window where she could at least sit and admire the stars.

Her fellow adoptee sister Eimy would be usually sitting and signing with her. Unfortunately, she was stuck in the ship's bowels, fixing one of the ship's engine filtration systems. United Earth Force had sent her to *Athena* as part of their ongoing efforts to consolidate their fleet for a more robust efficiency. *Athena* multi-tasked as a Hauler, a Science Vessel, and an occasional Emergency Towing Vessel.

The only other individual in Josephine's family who even attempted to learn any signs was their father. He tried, but he was always too busy being Captain. The best he could do was fingerspelling and signing the expletives. "Better than nothing" was a familiar, oft-repeated excuse. After all, everyone was too busy trying to keep up while mumbling annoyances at the new fleet-wide initiative. Josephine did understand, but she was still frustrated. It just wasn't enough.

Amidst the comets, asteroids, and the occasional planet, she sat alone and stared at the sparkling starry abyss.

Until Captain sat unexpectedly next to her. They admired the cosmos in silence. The unknown expanse, its celestial bodies: That was their language.

"Do you remember ..." he began to fingerspell, getting the letters "d" and "f" mixed up, "when we first met?"

How could she not? Seared into her nightmares was her upbringing in a penal colony that doubled as a shady adoption agency. She had been whisked away by nefarious agents looking to replenish their adoption agencies with fresh potential adoptees. Once kidnapped, Josephine was forced to dig holes. Just digging holes. A sea of unfamiliar faces masked the reason why she had to dig, and to this day she still didn't know why. She just knew she had to. When Captain and his team broke through to liberate the prisoners, she ran into his arms in a fit of gratitude. All the tears she had bottled up inside her poured out. It was then and there that he decided to adopt her.

Josephine gently tapped on her orb.

A virtual genderless avatar with an expressive face and in a black unitard appeared. With Josephine's press of a button, the avatar switched to Sign, smoothly interpreting Captain's voice and exasperated hands with near expert interpretation, except it was in the wrong sign language.

Josephine winced at the avatar, who was supposed to be fluent in Earth Sign Language. Her orb only knew the extinct American Sign Language. Ethan claimed that this was due to a system setting malfunction that couldn't be fixed before her arrival at *Athena*. *Oh, right,* she couldn't help wonder every time she used the orb. *Right.*

She had moaned many times to her father about how most of the crew had so little experience with EaSL. She sent out a memo to the crew with a hologram recording showing essential EaSL signs. EaSL was a constructed language that combined remnants of Indo-Pakistani Sign Language, Chinese Sign Language, Brazilian Sign Language, American Sign Language, and Plains Indian Sign Language. Sure, she could just use her avatar's Voice function, but not using the orb would be like spitting on the graves of those who had fought hard to resurrect Deaf culture.

EaSL traced its origins to a few native speakers who had survived the Great Purge of 2068. Hearing scientists, politicians, and educators had united to enact a combination of draconian policies to shut down Deaf schools and revoked accessibility accommodation laws in various countries such as the United States's Americans with Disabilities Act. Not only that, deafness was genetically modified out at birth; deafness-causing diseases were cured with a few simple tweaks of the person's core DNA sequence. For the Deaf community, it was another Dark Age. The holocaust of Deaf people was celebrated as a scientific triumph. Nobel Prizes were even awarded to these hearing scientific peers!

It wasn't until 2126, the year she was born, that people began to be born without auditory nerves. No one could correct this condition or figure out its cause. Not even a cochlear implant helped because there were no auditory nerves. For those born this way, their irises were a shade of emerald. These children watched old sign language videos preserved online and created EaSL. Eventually they resurrected the first Deaf club in almost a century by convening near the remains of Tower Clock, the only ruins left of the former Clerc-Gallaudet University. The Great Purge of 2068 had shut down the university along with ASL interpreter training programs across America. Amidst the ruins, these Deaf children established the linguistic foundation of EaSL.

"On this ship, I'm the goddamn Astrobiologist. I've studied the evolution of life beyond Earth," Josephine fumed to Captain. "Your son has me going through a never-ending holographic screens full of mumbo-jumbo. That's not what I've signed up for!" She stabbed at her food and wolfed down a bite. "Also," she voiced out loud, "he's a dick."

Everyone knew she hated using her deaf speech. And they knew that meant she was close to popping off like a stick of dynamite. The crew may not know her well, but they were very familiar with the infamous Kepler temper. That she wasn't biologically related to the Keplers didn't matter. She was a Kepler through and through.

Captain gave a placating gesture as curious eyes turned to watch.

"One more thing, Dad." She turned off her voice and flowed back to her hands, with the avatar punctuating her words. "I don't know what 'Molecular Disassembly' and 'Pattern Debigulators' means, or how to fuel 'Neural Implants of a Quantum-Secured Holographic Relocator.' My education did not include documenting clerical data of engineering mumbo-jumbo."

"I know," Captain sighed, cutting off her signing. "You're deaf, not dumb ..." He bloomed into a smile. "Also fierce. But you must try to empathize with Ethan's anxiety because this expedi—"

"Anxiety, my ass!" she cut off her father's words with a forceful wave.

"Josephine!" Captain tried to sign.

"Maybe if you had forced Ethan to follow up with my memo, give everyone a chance to get to know me, and learn some signs, too."

"Josephine!" Captain banged the table as he sternly fingerspelled her name, momentarily forgetting her sign name. It was one of the few signs he knew beyond the basic EaSL signs. "I recognize your efforts. Don't think I didn't notice that you've already implemented your new analysis module for bio-singles of alien lifeforms on this ship." He rubbed his eyes and pinched his nose in frustration. "I'll talk to Ethan about giving you more responsibility." He stood up. "But after this towing mission, though. We're still towing *Oïzús.*"

Before she could protest, he gave his sternest snarl that meant to convey intimidation, but she couldn't help but giggle. She'd seen him being a big softie one too many times.

This time he didn't smile. "Some electromagnetic field has been jamming our radio-galactic spectrum frequencies from *Oïzús,* and it's a dead ship?" He frowned. "We can't figure out where it's coming from. That's all I can say for now."

She nodded.

For a split second, she caught a genuine fear in his eyes, a rarity for someone who had always exuded a self-assured bravado. "I'm leading this one, and I promise I'll share the results with you. Just not right now."

He left, evidently believing that he'd said enough to placate her. *Oh, just another promise*, she thought. Another that would be broken when his duties as Captain eventually made him forget to create opportunities for the crew to learn some EaSL.

"Promises may get broken," she signed to her avatar as she flipped it off. "My spirit will never break ..."

She continued watching the wonders of the universe zoom past her window. Her orb buzzed and her sister Eimy's hologram appeared. Captions popped up below her chin. Sweat was caked on her skin, her braided pigtails undone as sweat stained her white, sleeveless tank top.

"Not going to be able—" the hologram glitched and warped, causing Josephine to miss what she even said. The text also became the dead language Eimy recognized as French. With a whack, the orb stopped malfunctioning. "Can you hear me now?"

Josephine flinched at the phrase. The man at the penal colony had gleefully mocked her with those words. She called him Kanuharmenuh as he sprayed septic water from a hose to keep her from being dehydrated in the mines. Her sister winced at her own accidental trigger.

"Shit!" Eimy cussed herself out. "I'm a fucking dumbass, I wasn't thinking. I was just saying I can't meet you for lunch." She disconnected, likely from embarrassment.

Accidents happened, Josephine knew, but sometimes she felt like that people intentionally triggered her tripwire with how frequently "accidents" happened.

She dropped off her tray and exited from the mess hall. She had evidently dumped the tray too hard, causing a loud noise, because everyone was staring at her. Ethan looked as if she'd pulled his pants down in front of everyone.

She shrugged and swiveled around to leave. Still, she bowed her head to ignore the sea of moving lips, laughter, and banter. She had tried to interact with these people in the past, but she learned that her crew mates put as much effort as she did into consuming her uneaten peas. They did try making small talk, but she'd keep asking, "What? What did you just say?" They responded with an awkward smile and said, "Oh, never mind." They had never felt comfortable with using her orb.

She tried to pretend their conversations were as bland as the ship's fluorescent, tubular halls. The 2130s ushered in the beigeification of intergalactic shuttles. Everything, right down to the toilet paper, was in

some shade of beige. Some space lobbyists convinced som
the Earth United Force that beige was neutrally safe for extra

"Not scientifically accurate," Josephine signed to he
sighing, pressing her palm on her entryway's keypad. Once in
she hopped onto her bed. "That prick," she signed when sh
about Ethan. Even the others handled her with kid gloves. *I*
token mascot, she thought.

She stared at the florescent tubes following the edges of the
They glowed a beige white indicating that all was fine upon the
The colors changed due to specific circumstances, mundane or
They used to announce such circumstances over the vessel's inter
but her arrival necessitated change. Captain wanted Josephine to
informed like the rest of the crew.

Josephine unscrewed the panels, pushed aside wires, and four
a dial with numbers. She had jerry-rigged the lighting to work as
flashing-light alarm for her without interfering with the ship's functions
She watched the tubes strobing around her room, lulling her to a blissful
sleep.

When her lights suddenly flashed yellow, she awoke. It was the
color of a shipwide emergency. She had napped longer than expected.
The intense flashing strained her eyes. She bolted up and scrambled
out of her room. She arrived at the airlocks, already crowded with crew
members, Captain's personal physician, and her siblings. Their faces
were aghast with fear.

She grabbed Eimy's shoulders for her attention. "What happ—"

Eimy hugged her fiercely, eyes swelling with tears. For once, Ethan
didn't look at her with scorn but with unbridled fear.

With a forceful elbow, Josephine escaped Eimy's embrace.

Some of the security muscleheads were fumbling with guns they
had barely used beyond training. Science Vessels rarely saw action. They
half-heartedly tried to stop her but they were freaking out.

Josephine saw what they saw: Captain. Her dad. He was slumped
against the elevator wall. Segments of his spine were slithering beneath
his skin. Each vertebra somehow looked like it was separated yet still
came across as aligned and attached to the spine. She saw the ebbs and
flows of skin, propelled by the vertebrae skittering underneath. Captain
was soaked in blood; he looked barely hanging on.

e generals in
terrestrials.
rself while
her room,
e thought
m just a

room.
essel.
dire.
om,
be

d
a

ad guard removed his helmet to
h syllable before his buddy punched

that Captain was covered with bits of his
seeped from his nose and ears, erupting
ace contorted in fear and his eyes drifted

er aside as the medic team collected him and
ridge crew following behind like nervous hens.
follow them, but Ethan stood in her way.
ned.

a hand, Ethan pulled his sister's interpreter orb rudely
et. Flicked it on. Even calibrated to the right settings.
ew how to use it.

shit," the avatar interpreted with an explosive emphasis.
dad. Not just yours. You're his midlife charity case. You've
logged his attention. You've been a drag on this family the
nt you arrived." He stepped forward, nearly blocking the hologram.
ologists. Otolaryngologists. Speech therapists. A rogue gallery of
tors." He shook his head, red in the face. "He missed my games.
our sister's events. He just had to take care of a broken, decrepit, and
attention-seeking whore."

No one moved. Within her peripheral vision, Josephine saw Eimy
clasping over her mouth.

He continued and turned his back to hide his face. "Maybe you
should cure yourself and not be a burden to people who can actually
contribute to society." He stomped away.

Josephine glanced at her sister who just stared gobsmacked.

She glanced down the hall slathered with a trail of red clashing with
the beige.

"Quarters, please. And I promise, Jo," Eimy grabbed her shoulders to
stave off interruption, "I'll tell you later."

Josephine stared down the hall. The unknown, every Deaf person's
biggest obstacle. Usually, she'd lipread. Find context clues within the
topic of relevance. Make educated guesses. But here was misplaced
anger. Chunks of flesh caked the floor along with the blood. *Screw later.*
She would find out now.

Once the coast was cleared, she kneeled down, taking keen note of the serrated cuts along what was left of a hand. The wounds appeared to be caused by a penetrating stylet appendage, perhaps from the extinct mosquito. Had someone illegally revived the species?

She glanced back toward the elevator. She boarded it for the docking bay where the investigative team were scrutinizing the away team's shuttle for damages. It was battered and bloodied; some parts were still aflame. Ethan's team were taking forensic samples.

Bobbing and weaving around in between people and storage containers, she walked like she belonged there. She knew no one would bug one of Captain's kids. She quickly hid behind the second-to-last storage unit near the docking bay's door. Two figures emerged in blue hazmat suits. They carried out a green cadaver bag.

I must see the footage, she thought, not daring to sign and risk capturing attention. She slipped past them through the door and immediately halted at the grisly scene before her.

One of the cadaver bags was unzipped. A corpse was face down with their back blown out. The ribs flared upward and outward with organs either sagging like raisins on the floor or hanging like ornaments off the mangled ribs. Despite her extreme disgust, she noticed a peculiar detail: No spine.

She shimmied herself into an oversized cabinet. For once, being petite came in handy. The hazmat suits returned and somberly marched out. She stumbled out, nearly losing her balance, and proceeded to type away on the shuttle's viewscreen by the door. A glowing titanium cylinder popped out a holographic disc containing footage from the ship's outer security camera.

With whatever the hell was going on, Josephine knew being told later might not even happen. She moved quickly past the pandemonium and headed for her room.

Locking her door, she slid the disc into her holographic projector. The screen opened to the deserted corridors of *Oïzús*, the ship that Athena was towing home. She scrub-forwarded through the footage. No sign of life anywhere. Very eerie. Then suddenly, she saw all twenty members of the away team exit from the shuttle. Her father was pointing, taking charge while being shadowed by two hulking members of security. No one looked scared or confused, but there was a sense of urgency. She knew her father would bring some of the best out in his crew to save whoever was in distress.

As the away team exited offscreen, she steeled herself as she watched derelict exhaust pipes, clearly ripped from the walls, discharging toxic fumes. The ashen discharge morphing into steam flowed into the air like lava. She noted the tiny organisms attempting to salvage the ruined ship into a new ecosystem. One she knew she'd never get the privilege to explore. Eventually, she found the courage to scrub-forward the footage until she saw a body get flung away violently at a high speed. The tangled mass of human limbs barely quivered with life as a sea-green emerald gelatin mucus covered the crew member.

She scrub-backwarded the disc and flicked on her neuron analyzer, a device that could instantly analyze the neurons of all biologicals appearing on the screen. She paused on the clearest pixelation of the organism in spite of the electromagnetic interference. By judging how fast actions the organism moved, crucial data could be extrapolated. For example, before the crewmate was flung, an intense aquamarine hue flashed, blinding the camera. It lasted no longer than ten nanoseconds. Actually, 300 picoseconds, according to her own sensor's calculations. This new organism had the potential of unleashing a force that mirrored a shotgun blaster.

Which explained the bits.

She zoomed onto the organism's appendage and then pulled back. Its face had a birdlike shape covered with helix spirals that repeated in an exquisite pattern while its vibrissae was surrounded by stiff hairs.

The reading indicated that its vibrissae was producing a phenomenon rare to occur in any known biological organism: sonoluminescence. The sensors indicated that the creature's extremity had an organic gelatine core that reached temperatures of over 4,700 degrees Celsius.

Oh, my God, Josephine thought as she realized the extremity was more like a pistol as she watched another rescue crew member get annihilated with its bioacoustical blast that cooked the victim into a liquid carnage. The creature glowed a neon green before it commenced with another round of blasts at someone else out of the frame.

She held her breath as she saw her father and his security guards hauling ass back to the ship, not realizing that they were entering the belly of—*what? It needs a name*, Josephine thought. A name always cast a light into the unknown. It gave fear a face. She paused the screen, eyeing the creature more carefully. She noted the helical patterns on the various masses floating within its gelatin body. This creature's stance reminded her of the red kangaroo, an extinct unipedal mammal. The striking ever-changing green hues that colored the gelatin substance in its body inspired her with its new name. *The prevalence of Helix shapes, cylindrical spirals ... if I borrow the Greek's definition of "green" with Chloro ...* Josephine spoke and signed aloud a name: "Helichloros!"

The helichloros glowed, its blasters turning luminous as a bright explosion shot out at her father, who fell to his knees as he held his ears in agony. The helichloros thrust its prehensile tail at him, spewing its mucus onto him. Just as the creature dug into his neck, he was dragged offscreen.

With what looked like a sickly thump, the Captain fell, clawing at the floor as he was dragged off screen. The guard who was with him fired back at the helichloros but he dropped to his knees, clutching his helmet in apparent agony. Another glow offscreen before she exhaled: His head was gone.

Frantically, she scrub-forwarded the disc until she saw Captain limping back to the shuttle. The timestamp showed three hours had eclipsed. He staggered along, hunched over with his spine's segments slithering underneath his skin like beetles. The movement with the scrub-forward made them wiggle even more creepily.

The screen blinked to red, along with the tubular lights in her room. Both began flashing red: *Crimson Alert.* This meant an ongoing emergency with casualties. "Shit," she signed, grabbing her spare orb. She would do what her dad would always say at the end of every mission: "Blow this popsicle stand."

She click-opened her door and collided into Eimy who winced but promptly locked her door, sealing them from whatever hellish nightmare out there.

Collapsing on her bed, Eimy clutched her head as blood poured out of her ears. Josephine held her sister as she screamed in despair.

"I'm here, Eimy," she held her, whispering to her ears. "I'm here. I'm here." Eimy lay there, sobbing on the bed. What the helichloros did hadn't seemed to affect her like it did Eimy. Her deafness must've neutralized the effects of bioacoustical blasting from the creature. *It's all sound waves,* Josephine thought.

She flicked her avatar on and began furiously signing. "Stay here! You're safe." She unclicked the door while signing with the other hand. "I'm going to save our prick of a brother, then we go to the escape pods." Eimy grabbed her arm with sheer panic in her eyes begging her to stay.

Josephine broke free as Eimy exclaimed, "There's these ... these ..." she stifled herself with a cry.

Josephine hit *eject* on the projector, grabbed the hologram disc, and lobbed it at her sniffling sister.

"Is that what I think it is?" Eimy asked.

Josephine nodded. "I'm Deaf, not stupid."

"Wait a minute." Eimy perked up. "You must be immune. Since you weren't squirming on the floor with me ..."

Josephine smiled. "We need a plan. I need to gather up my orbs."

"Why?"

"You never know."

"Really? What are you proposing?"

Josephine explained her plan, and Eimy nodded with pride.

Not even a minute later, they bolted from the room. Josephine retrieved a blaster from a dead guard. His hand was still clasped onto the pistol grip. Together the sisters peeled his fingers off the weapon, which Josephine grabbed.

Eimy ran with her as best she could while they tried to avert their eyes from the carnage surrounding them.

Josephine dropped low and slid across the smooth floor as she fired point blank shots at the helichloros about to blast at her sister. She turned to the next monster and fired. Both creatures collapsed.

Up close, the dead helichloroses were indeed a sight to behold. Their skin appeared to be a calcium-collagen hide, a sickly violet skin with vibrissae that seemed to function as vibrating hairs. *They must be using their hairs as sort of an echolocational function*, Josephine thought. *But just how—*

Then another helichloros suddenly pounced from the shadows and tried to blast at Josephine. Due to their sluggish movements, she was able to roll out of the way in time. *They must be using sonic attacks to immobilize their prey*, she thought. She felt the force of their 62 miles an hour attack brush past her. Dodging one slow helichloros is one thing, but a dozen helichloroses blasting at once? The odds were obviously in their favor. She fired at the next helichloros's cranium and looked up at her sister as she pumped her blaster, checking to see if her gun had cooled enough. An overheated gun would be useless.

"Ethan's staying with Dad in the med bay."

"Let's go save the prick."

The sisters leaped to their feet and turned the corner toward the elevator for the med bay. As they rode the elevator down, they finally took a breath.

Unfortunately, they had their breaths taken away when the elevator opened to the sight of a horde of helichloroses, their spiral, empty pseudoeyes staring absentmindedly at them as they blocked the entry way to the med bay.

A detached arm was left on the floor right in front of the elevator. The sisters stared slack-jawed.

"Oops," gasped Eimy as she hit the emergency alarm button, and slowly the door closed.

The sisters jumped apart from the impact of their blasts as the door closed. A big dent radiated smoke from their onslaught of blasts. They knew that sooner or later, the Helichloros would burst through the elevator door.

"Shit!" Eimy turned to her. "Any bright ideas?"

She grabbed Eimy, forcefully shimmying her right up to the elevator door and barely shielding her from the creatures' line of fire.

"Don't. Move."

Josephine pressed the button to reopen the door. She flicked on her orb and lobbed it down the hallway. It rolled and landed a ways from the entrance to the med bay.

The HoloInterpreter bloomed into life and began to SimCom an ancient Earth classic about two cities: "It was the best of times, it was the worst of times ..." Their attention diverted, the horde began to prowl closer to the hologram. Their bodies became lit: unmerry Christmas lights. When the orb's blinding light dimmed, the creatures all lunged through the hologram.

The sisters ran like they never ran before. They slipped and skidded over the ruptured bodies and puddles of blood.

Then a few helichloroses slowly shifted toward them.

They glanced at each other. Both realized a cold, hard fact.

What if no one was on the other side? They held each other's hands and closed their eyes, bracing for the end. With her deafness, Josephine knew she had a viable chance to escape, but that would've meant doing the unthinkable: leaving her sister to be slaughtered.

Ethan unceremoniously opened the door and pulled them inside. "They would leave eventually, but nooo, you both had—" he shushed up as they rushed into him with hugs. "I'm sorry," he mouthed as he looked over at their father's corpse. Even covered with a thick blanket, one could see the shape of his protruding ribs.

"*I'm sorry,*" Ethan signed with an emphasis to Josephine.

"You can't take back the words," she sadly signed. "But 'sorry' is a start. We need to go."

Ethan smiled grimly. "We're safe here. Eventually they'll leave ..."

The sisters looked unconvinced as they gazed back through the triple-paned window at the helichloroses standing still as Komainu statues. He took the last spare orb from Josephine's lab coat and flicked it on.

"If we listen to you, we'll end up dead. Naturally being Captain's son, I'm—"

Eimy slapped him into silence and yelled, "If you don't listen to her, I'm going to connect my steel-toed boots up your candy ass."

He said, "How is she going to hea—"

She shoved him back, grabbed a rifle off the wall next to them, and handed it to Josephine. "Ethan, pick one. Still will connect boot to ass." She grabbed a gauze rope off a nearby shelf, and tied it around herself and Ethan's waists. "She's immune to their sonic attacks." She pointed to the makeshift gauze rope she was tying into knots. "Keep following where she tugs us even if they're immobilizing. And we need to muffle our ears for protection." She stuffed pieces of gauze into their ears.

"I'm an ass, not a dumbass," he said as he tested the knot that tied to him, "You're telling me she—" he hooked a thumb at Josephine "—can withstand the sound frequency of 196 kHz with an intensity of 10 W/cm²?" He laughed out the last bit with every ounce of fundamental scorn possible. "A calculated 218 decibels that's decimating us all?!"

In unison the sisters signed, "*Yes.*"

As the door opened, they dragged him as Josephine flung her last orb past the creatures. The second avatar flared to life and resumed the

Holobook from before. The creatures remained unfazed, revving up their blasters which glowed, but their skin remained dim.

"Shit, shit, shit, shit," Ethan cried. "They're not mindless killing machines." The helichloroses had deciphered their strategy already.

Josephine fired a barrage of plasma bolts to confuse the creatures away. The trio ran into the cleared path back into the elevator and pushed the button for the fourth floor. A tangle of limbs, they helped each other up to their feet and braced themselves as the door opened to the corridor leading to the escape pods. They were relieved to find the blood-splattered corridor empty.

Eimy and Ethan followed their duel-wielding sister and suddenly tugged her to a halt. They had heard a helichloros skittering above them on the ceiling. Its slimy sea green mucus dripped down upon them. Its head was twitching with anticipation.

All three stood in pregnant silence, not daring to move or breathe.

Josephine lined her gun up at the creature, but Ethan pushed her gun away. He wagged his finger no and motioned to his sisters to follow him.

The trio slowly reached one of the last remaining pods. As Eimy searched near the door for the flight initiation lever to prepare the pod, Ethan collapsed in front of their pod.

"Ggggaaaaaarrrrgh," he moaned.

The sisters caught sight of a wound at the bottom of his neck on the back over his spinal cord.

Meanwhile the helichloros began vibrating its body. Its skin hummed its now familiar glow. Its helical false eyes swayed with intensity. Its purple segments tremored like the tail of a Texan rattler.

Eimy's eyes widened as Josephine took a rifle and double-tapped plasma pellets right into its skull as it lunged forward with an unexpected speed; it must've coiled in all its energy before springing. Its tail buoyed itself as if it was a kangeroo. Its blood splattered everywhere, leaving a metallic purple sheen next to Josephine's feet.

Josephine attended to Ethan, ripping the back of his shirt, as each of his vertebrae began to wiggle and squirm out of place. Soon, she knew, his vertebrae would be swimming around inside his back like their father's.

Contorted with grief, Eimy pulled her sister into the pod.

Josephine shook off her attempts, looking confusedly at both of them. "What?" She still stood outside the pod.

"I'll be okay," Ethan pleaded as he tried to turn and hide his back. "I'm not leaving this ship." He tried to smile through the pain.

Eimy glanced around and spotted the flight initiation lever. Without preamble she pulled it to boot up the escape pod. The flight initiation sequence would not take long before they took off.

Ethan quickly turned and trembled from whatever sound he was hearing. They all saw a very faint green hue.

The helichloros they had killed had summoned its friends.

"Ethan," Josephine kneeled, Sim-Commed, "we can figure this out. Haul ass. Now!"

"The human body has 33 vertebrae," Ethan said. "Do the math. I did."

Josephine's eyes widened with understanding.

"It has to end on this ship. Which means, I must stay." With a brittle smile, he grabbed one of the blasters. "At least allow me to die like a hero."

Josephine rolled her eyes. "Guess you're not such a prick after all, eh?" But she didn't give him a chance to respond when she abruptly hugged him.

Then Eimy mournfully but playfully shoved him away from their pod. "Be a hero before you ruin the moment."

The three hugged together.

"Will you both be all right?" Ethan asked.

She wanted to say, "I'll tell you later," but chose instead to use the classic ASL handshape sign for "I love you."

Eimy pulled her sister inside the pod as the outer door sealed shut.

Josephine avoided looking through their window, ignoring Eimy's attempts to muffle the sound of their brother's screams as his vertebrae slowly began to break-emerge despite his attempts to look heroic.

As the pod began to disconnect from the ship, a light show of plasma erupted. The white light illuminated the inside of the pod. It faded as the last shot was fired.

Meanwhile Josephine was already looking to the future, wondering, *What did Dad know about the Helichloros on Oïzús?* Hadn't there been occasional snippeted reports of a mysterious creature appearing unbidden on other ships? She would have to investigate once they landed on Earth. If she herself was indeed immune to the sonic blasts from the helichloroses, it would make sense that she and other Deaf people together could eradicate the mysterious creature. Perhaps she might finally earn the respect long overdue to the Deaf community.

Is That It?

I grew up in a farming family in the west of Ireland, where my family worked hard to earn a living from the farm. I was sent to a boarding school in Cabra, Dublin, where I shared meals with other Deaf boys at the dinner table. However, the school strictly forbade the use of sign language. We were taught using the oral system by hearing teachers, but I secretly used sign language with a group of boys, careful not to be caught. Typically, I was sent home every second weekend, as well as during Christmas, St. Patrick's Day, Easter, and for two months over the summer holidays.

I came home to see my family every second weekend. At the dinner table, my father always sat at the center. I found it difficult to participate in conversations; my father and mother spoke at a pace that was impossible for me to follow, and understanding their words was a constant struggle. While I could grasp what my father was saying, my mother's rapid speech often left me frustrated. She frequently scolded me, and I tended to ignore her remarks. Instead, I communicated with my youngest sister, who was more attuned to my needs. I don't fully understand why, but I had a strong bond with her. It was easier for me to follow her lipreading and gestures.

After my father's death, our family grew with the addition of my brother and baby sister. As they grew older, they joined the rest of us at the dinner table, where I sat at the head along with my mother and siblings. Whenever I came home on weekends and we gathered for dinner, I could see my family engaged in conversation, which often left me feeling disconnected as I struggled to follow their spoken words. Every morning, either my mother or my sister would listen to the radio, which brought us news of daily life in the west of Ireland. My mother frequently informed me about local deaths and upcoming funerals. Similarly, my sister would share news that she knew would interest me, such as the unexpected death of a famous movie star, knowing my love for both classic and modern films.

One morning at breakfast table, when my sister heard breaking news on the radio, I asked her what it was about. She told me to wait a moment, saying, "I'll tell you later." I waited patiently while she continued to listen, and eventually, she shared bits of information about the IRA bombings in Northern Ireland. This conflict between Catholics and Protestants has been ongoing since the 1970s. When she gave me only a brief update about where the bomb was located and how many were killed, I responded, "Is that it? No more information?" My sister only had a little more to share about the incident. Later that evening, I watched the news on TV, which showed video footage of the bombings in Northern Ireland that my sister had mentioned earlier in the day. Interestingly, TV stations in Ireland lacked subtitles until they were introduced in 1991.

During the 1980s, I was a teenager that time my cousin graciously invited me to a wedding reception held at a hotel. It was my first time attending my cousin's wedding. Over 100 guests attended, enjoying a three-course meal. The tables were beautifully set with sparkling white linen, small vases of wildflowers in the center, and unfortunately, the glare from silver brass candlelight. Round tables, which are typically conducive to conversation for Deaf people, were present. However, it was a predominantly hearing crowd. I attended with my mother, her close male friend, and my sister. While my family engaged in conversation easily, I found it difficult to follow along. I pretended to be comfortable, masking my discomfort with a fake smile, trying to appear as though I belonged at the dinner table. It was a challenge; I felt isolated and unable to participate in their conversations, missing out on the opportunity to catch up on the day-to-day news they shared. It was daunting to deal with my hearing family and cousins at such gatherings. I found it easier to have one-on-one conversations rather than trying to keep up with the lively discussions of the larger group.

I often visited my relatives' homes for dinner invitations or anniversary celebrations at hotels or restaurants. Sometimes, it was just a normal dinner where I could engage in one-on-one conversations, making it easier to follow along more frequently. Typically, at these gatherings, spoken language dominated. As the only Deaf person among hearing families on every occasion, I sometimes felt lonely. The hearing family members' lack of knowledge about sign language had a significant impact on my life. Not many were fully aware of the challenges a Deaf person faces at the dinner table, often leaving me feeling excluded and isolated during these lengthy conversations.

My uncle or aunt always asks, "How is your life in Dublin?"

I usually respond with, "It's fine, and life in Dublin is busy."

I briefly mention my job and daily life, but the conversations are limited. I set boundaries on the depth of these discussions. However, when I meet my close cousin, we often have longer conversations about what's happening in our lives. I don't know why, but I feel more comfortable talking with my close cousin, who seems to understand me better than my aunt and uncle do. It's strange how limited my conversations are with my other hearing family members.

As I entered my adult years and left home, I no longer had regular dinner gatherings with my family or relatives. Instead, I joined the Deaf community for various celebrations such as dinner dances, parties, weddings, christenings, and funerals. At these events, I found myself among many Deaf individuals, all of us gathering around round tables for meals. We shared in sign language, grateful for the round tables that allowed us to see each other clearly—a more suitable arrangement than square tables. I appreciate the manufacturers of these round tables, which facilitate easier communication for Deaf people. At these gatherings, there was no need to say, "I will tell you later." We shared a common sense of understanding and equality, communicating solely through sign language instead of spoken language, unlike our interactions with hearing family, colleagues, and associates.

For me, growing up involved navigating two distinct worlds: the hearing and Deaf communities, which are fundamentally different. The two cultures diverge significantly; in the Deaf community, people tend to be very blunt and straightforward, whereas the hearing community might find such directness sensitive or jarring. This difference in communication styles often becomes apparent during gatherings like dinner parties. I noticed that the members of the Deaf community might not realize how their approach can come across as resistant or unsettling to hearing individuals, who might be hesitant to speak out. These dynamics are especially noticeable at the dinner table during special occasions such as award ceremonies, festivals, and weddings

In the 1990s, I joined the hearing world when I started working at a clothing warehouse with about twenty hearing individuals. I was the only Deaf person among the hearing staff. Normally, I conversed with the hearing staff one-on-one. The staff had a good attitude and were very respectful. They were aware that I was Deaf, so most of our conversations involved lipreading or gesturing. This allowed me to befriend them and share meaningful conversations about various issues and news. However, during the fifteen-minute breaks and one hour lunch, I joined the hearing staff at a large table in the spacious kitchen. Trying to keep up with the conversations at the table proved quite impossible, so I would often ask one of the staff members what everyone was talking about. They would give me a brief summary of the day's news. I was often disappointed that the updates were minimal, much like the conversations with my hearing family at home. This was a significant impact on my life, highlighting the challenges of conversing with the hearing staff. I knew that the hearing staff enjoyed lively discussions about daily news and shared funny stories or jokes. However, the humor from the hearing staff, which often involved Irish jokes common during breaks, was lost on me. I found it hard to follow their words, which did not resonate with Deaf humor that relies heavily on facial expressions, body language, and sign language. Sometimes I felt left out by the hearing staff at the table because I had no interest in following their conversations. Instead, I would go for a walk or shop for an hour, which didn't bother me at all.

In the Deaf community, we often refer to ourselves as one family when we share stories and experiences of the oppression we face when our hearing families do not use sign language.

RAYMOND LUCZAK

The Moment When I Died

The moment when I died was the first time I understood everything I'd misunderstood for so long I wanted to head back and apologize and make amends.

My entire life became a reel that spun a million revolutions per second, and yet everything was crystal clear, as if in slow motion.

It was surreal to see myself as a little girl, and to see my body metamorphosing into that of a young woman. Did I really look like her?

I had been so long accustomed to seeing myself as an old woman that the shock of seeing so much youth in her face, in her movements, lingered for a long time afterward, filtering through the spectacle of middle age when my son Derek sneered at me. "You're not a good mother, Mom. You never were."

Oh, how those words hurt.

The way his nasal speech, emptied of most consonants, had echoed over and over again in my dreams. How could he make such a vile accusation? Hadn't I toiled so hard to make sure that all our kids were fed? What a selfish thing to say after all I'd done for him!

No matter how much I'd prayed to God for intervention, my son refused to return for even a short visit.

Five years later, I died.

The moment when I died was the first time I realized how different my new world would become after traveling three hours to have Derek's hearing tested in an audiology clinic at the university. Jim and I had suspicions that Derek had a hearing problem, but we weren't sure. He didn't seem to know his name when we called him to dinner. His doctor suggested that we get his hearing tested.

Our appointment was with Mr. Wevill, an older audiologist who was due to retire at any moment. Something about his casual suit and loosened tie made me feel that I could trust him.

In the big glassed-in room, Derek fidgeted on a small chair. A small number of plush toys covered with loud colors distracted him. It was tough to test his hearing. He didn't seem to understand that he was supposed to raise his hand each time he heard a sound in his headphones. He also tried to push the headphones off his head. A young woman, who was a graduate student in the audiology department, sat patiently with him, trying to redirect his attention to the sounds that were beeping into his ears.

Watching Derek and the young woman while sitting next to Mr. Wevill as he rotated his dials and notated the X's and O's across Derek's first audiogram chart, I felt like a mass of nerves with nowhere to go but everywhere to scream. How I wanted him to raise his hand!

But I kept my face calm as porcelain. I would not show anyone the storm of emotions ranging inside me. After all, I was his mother, and he needed to know who was in charge.

I was so relieved when the woman finally brought Derek back into Mr. Wevill's office. He ran right into my arms. I almost cried.

Then came the diagnosis. After looking quickly at the audiogram, Mr. Wevill said, "Well, looks like he's profoundly deaf. Derek's gonna need hearing aids."

I inhaled. I would not cry.

Derek wasn't even two years old. He seemed to have forgotten already having worn headphones. I immediately held him close to my chest. "How's he going to survive?" I didn't know that I would hug him differently than any of my five other kids.

I fell into a blur of worrying about Derek's future and taking him back to Mr. Wevill, another three-hour trip each way, when his first pair of earmolds came in, and I watched him trying to pull them out.

Mr. Wevill sighed and used a nail file to narrow down the earmold's thickness so it could fit better inside his ear.

Then Derek pulled out both of his earmolds and unbuckled his hearing aid, which was bulky and rechargeable. He threw everything onto the floor.

My heart stopped. "Derek!"

The audiologist chuckled. "He doesn't understand why he's supposed to wear them. Hold on a sec." He pulled out a binder from a shelf near his desk. There were pictures of young kids wearing hearing aids. He brought it down to Derek and pointed to the pictures. "These. Are deaf kids. You. Look. This is you!"

Derek stared at the pictures for a full minute. He had never stopped to stare at anything for long. He was always glancing around, looking.

"But ..."

"Shhh," Mr. Wevill said. "He has to feel that it's all up to him."

Derek glanced back at the floor where his hearing aid was. He picked it up and looked at it. He turned it around and around. It was clear that it didn't look like the same hearing aids that the deaf children wore in the pictures.

Mr. Wevill bent down to the floor and pulled up the earmolds by their cords. He directed Derek's eyes back to the picture and pointed to the deaf children's ears. Every one of them was wearing earmolds with cords attached to their hearing aids solidly in front of their small chests.

A few minutes later Mr. Wevill was able to put the earmolds back into Derek's ears and adjusted the straps containing his first hearing aid. He looked directly into Derek's eyes and pointed to his hearing aid.

When Derek looked down at his hearing aid, Mr. Wevill tapped the top of it gently.

Derek looked at me, startled. It was the first sound he heard clearly using a hearing aid.

I was never prouder of him than in that moment.

The moment when I died was the first time I sat down with Mrs. Niller, Derek's new speech therapist. She was among the many young and eager women I'd meet over the years when it came to his education, and I liked her right off the bat. Nothing seemed to faze her, and she laughed easily.

I brought Derek to an empty classroom at an elementary school not far from where we lived. Classes had been dismissed for the day, but Mrs. Niller was willing to start Derek early on his speech therapy. He was still too young to go to school.

By then Derek had seemed to accept his hearing aid. His brothers and sisters found his hearing aid to be weird, but in time they stopped saying anything about it. Derek strapped it onto his chest like most people with bad vision would put on their glasses at the start of the day. I couldn't always tell if he heard anything, but there were times when I saw a flicker of puzzlement when he heard something new and different, like a sharp caw from across the street.

I tried to tell him. "You just heard a crow. Over there." I rushed him to the front window where our street was lined with tall trees where crows liked to perch. He still looked confused when I pointed up to the trees and tried to explain. It was clear on his face that he understood he was quite different from us.

At the school, Mrs. Niller opened a full-color book that had words set in bold type beneath each illustration.

Derek sat next to me as she pointed to each picture. "Man," she said. "Woman."

"Boy."

"Girl."

"Dog."

"Cat."

But he didn't seem to understand what he was supposed to do.

"Come over here," she said.

Derek walked around the table to her.

"Now," she said. "Just feel this." She took his hand and brought it up to her throat. "Bum-bum-bum!"

He stopped, then looked at me.

I pointed to my own throat and said, "Bum-bum-bum!"

She repeated, "Bum-bum-bum!"

He opened his mouth and tried to make movements.

She whipped out a small mirror and held it up to their faces close together. "Look. Bum-bum-bum!"

She brought his hand to her throat, then to his own.

His first utterance sounded so timid. "Bub-bub-bub."

"Yes! You got it!"

She and I looked at each other with glee.

"Bub-bub-bub! Bub-bub-bub!"

He was such a good student that I didn't fear that he'd try to learn sign language.

The moment when I died was the first time I was forced to wonder whether it was fair to any of my kids to be part of a large family.

My husband Jim was often too tired to do anything when he got home from the warehouse. He worked six days a week, not five, because he needed the extra money to help pay for the house and the kids. He had wanted to have a large family, but I don't think he'd understood just how expensive that was going to be.

I didn't understand at the time how large families can exact a terrible price that has nothing to do with money. No child gets enough individual attention. Someone always gets left behind.

The moment when I died was the first time I realized that the town where I grew up wasn't big enough to provide the education Derek needed. I didn't want him to move away for months at a time where he'd live downstate at a Deaf residential school. I didn't want him to turn into a stranger.

Mrs. Niller said that he was learning new words all the time, and more than that, he was *retaining* them. He remembered how to pronounce the new words correctly. He was even learning how to read sentences.

He gradually learned how to speak English. He still mispronounced some words. Most of his consonants were missing, but he was still understandable.

Each time he spoke clearly and naturally, it felt like a cause for celebration.

I now understand that during those days, my son began to wonder about me. Why wasn't I paying attention to him like before?

I was so busy with cooking and feeding and washing clothes and taking the kids to the doctor and dentist that I eventually stopped paying as much attention to Derek as I had before.

He still spoke as before, but it'd never occurred to me that he wasn't part of the happy babble around the table at mealtimes. No one paid attention to him.

When I allow myself to *really* look at his face at those times in the reel of my life, I feel a stab in my heart. It really hurts.

The moment when I died was the first time Jim and I brought Derek to his foster family who lived two hours away from home but close to a speech program for deaf kids. The new town was almost the same as mine, but it was more centrally located for other deaf kids in the region. They, too, would stay with foster families.

The Sundays seemed like a nice family. Mr. Sunday was the vice principal at the local high school, and Mrs. Sunday was a part-time teacher's aide who worked with disabled kids at Derek's new elementary school. Their three kids had all grown up and gone away. Mrs. Sunday said that she would pick him up every day after school, and she was glad to take care of him. She wasn't a grandmother yet, but she was eager to get started on her grandmothering.

Leaving him with the Sundays was the hardest decision of my life. I felt ripped in half. I didn't know if I could trust such strangers like that. I didn't understand that he would inevitably compare his foster family with our family and wonder why we couldn't be the same. Jim held my hand while I cried on our way back home.

Because Derek was the only child in their house, he got the attention he craved. There were only the three of them at mealtime. Sometimes their adult kids would visit from out of town, but Mrs. Sunday was quite emphatic about them looking directly at Derek each time they spoke.

In those days, long-distance calls were very expensive. Mrs. Sunday wrote newsy letters to me every week, which she gave to Derek to give to me.

I didn't understand how it was possible for her to say that he was such a bright and happy boy because when he came home with a college student every weekend, he seemed a bit listless. Was he really happy up there? Or was Mrs. Sunday lying to me in order to make me feel better about leaving Derek alone with them?

The moment when I died was the first time I felt quiet jolts of pride when Janey Mitchell, who lived down the street from us, remarked, "Your son's doing real well. I can tell. He speaks so good!"

That gave me hope.

I couldn't wait for him to come home every Friday, and I didn't want him to leave every Sunday afternoon.

His weekly absences left a hole that I pretended didn't exist. Having to take care of a house filled with my other five kids and a husband helped some, but not much.

*

The moment when I died was the first time I finally understood why Derek had become so angry.

The more he learned to speak, the more he asked me what was going on at the dinner table. The banter was rapid-fire. I couldn't keep up, but I couldn't stop laughing. My kids were so funny!

I didn't know that the most toxic four words for a deaf kid in a hearing household with no signing were "I'll tell you later."

Even more damning were the equally toxic four words "I'm sorry I forgot."

Those years when all of the kids lived at home went by like a blur, and I hadn't realized how often I said those words. Over and over again.

And yet we expected him to sit there and pretend he was able to follow the jokes leapfrogging all over the table.

Over and over *again*.

And yet we wanted to believe that he was such an expert lipreader that he didn't need any help at mealtime. The fact that none of us had ever wondered why he never laughed with us horrifies me now. I have no physical body of my own now, but if I did, it would've been filled with the hot fire of shame.

The moment when I died was the first time when Derek, now a full-grown man, came home for Christmas after his first semester away at college. I didn't want him to attend Gallaudet because it was full of Deaf people who signed, but it was the only college he wanted to attend. He was among the very few students who had scored a full four-year scholarship. I was so proud of him that I wanted to frame that letter congratulating him on the scholarship.

Seeing him leave our house again for college tore me up all over again. I didn't want him to leave. And Washington, DC, was a big city! How was he going to cope?

That December when he returned, the changes in him were startling and frightening. He was no longer quiet. He sported a full beard. He wore a T-shirt and an old tweed jacket he found in a thrift shop. He was upfront about using sign language even when he used his voice. He made sure that his presence was felt. He demanded to know what *all* of us were saying. None of us knew what to do, what to make of him.

I didn't understand that we'd expected him to stay quiet in the background, the way he always was at the dinner table. I didn't understand that the point of college was not to earn a degree. College was supposed to encourage independent thinking.

I hadn't grasped how independently Derek had been thinking all those years when he lived at home. Growing up, he just didn't know the words to describe those thoughts then. Being among other Deaf people his age gave him the confidence that I hadn't realized I didn't want him to have after all. He wasn't alone with his feelings.

I didn't like thinking about sign language. It was too distracting. It meant that the user was a speech failure.

My son had excellent speech! Why was he so adamant about using ASL? Why did he feel like he had to make a political statement with everything he said? Couldn't he be quiet and normal like before?

Why was he throwing away all those years he'd spent learning how to speak clearly?

I didn't appreciate his ingratitude.

The moment when I died was the first time I turned down the one chance I had to reconnect with Derek. The local community college had been offering ASL classes, and since I was officially a senior citizen, I was eligible to take the class for free.

Derek insisted that I go. "It's free!"

I shook my head no. "My hands are too stiff now. My fingers. See?" I showed him how I was developing arthritis in my hands. Which wasn't exactly true. It just looked too complicated for me. I didn't want to feel stupid.

He said, "You can adapt. I even know a Deaf guy who has only one hand. It's not a problem for him. We understand him just fine."

"Nah," I said. "Too much work."

I didn't catch how he nearly bit his own lip.

I wouldn't realize until after I'd died that that was the moment he began to question seriously why he had bothered to come home and visit with me and Jim in the first place. He had spent many years learning how to speak with us, but I couldn't be bothered to learn how to sign a few things?

It would be a few years before I saw him again.

The moment when I died was the last time I saw him leave my house. Jim had died the year before, so Derek had come to spend a weekend with me. He had been recently promoted to a new job that involved data analysis at some corporation. I never understood exactly what he did for a living, but it paid well.

In the beginning, we talked easily. He wanted to know what was up with each of his siblings and their kids.

At the kitchen table we talked and talked about relatives who'd died a long time before.

I told him stories that I hadn't realized he never heard before because he couldn't follow the family babble at the dinner table years ago.

Then we fell into a horrible argument. I had said that I was surprised he didn't know the story about Uncle Harry and his first wife's death.

He said, "How would I know? Everybody was yakking at the same time!" He paused. "Hearing people are selfish, period."

That set me off. I explained that we hearing people didn't have to help deaf people like him learn how to speak, but we did anyway. That I didn't understand what he'd truly meant would become the biggest regret of my life.

"Really? I can't believe you said that. As if you're doing me a *fucking* favor!"

The crude language shocked me. "Don't you dare use—"

"You're not a good mother, Mom. You never were."

"What?"

"You could've told everyone to stop talking all at once! Set up rules for talking at the table."

"I can't—"

"No. You could've, but you didn't want to. You didn't feel you could tell us kids how to behave, but you. *Could*. Have! But you didn't. I don't feel close to my brothers and sisters because they don't take the time to talk to me! I'm too much work."

"Derek—"

"You know how things could've been better? Because when I stayed with the Sundays, they always made sure I understood everything at the table! It's not hard."

"But when you've got five kids—"

"You and Dad were the *adults*. You didn't tell them to stop and listen! I'm so, *so* tired of hearing people making excuses when they should know better. Nobody *listens* in this family! I'm done." He left the kitchen.

"Wait—"

But it was too late. I heard him storm upstairs to his old room where he stayed for a while.

I figured that he had needed to calm down for a bit.

I didn't know it then, but he was packing his suitcase and texting for a cab ride to a motel.

I sat in the living room, trying to watch some TV.

Then I heard his footsteps go down the stairs and leave through the kitchen and the side door outside.

Then I heard a car park in front of my house.

I hurried to the front window and peered through the curtain.

He didn't look back at the house as he got into the cab.

It was the last time I would see him while I was still alive.

The moment when I died was the first time I felt so painfully helpless without Jim. He had always comforted me when I went on and on about Derek. "He'll come around," he said. "Just give him time."

Then I told my kids about the awful things Derek had said.

They said, "You're a great mother. You really took care of us!"

They agreed that Derek had anger management issues. "Why does being deaf have to be such a big deal? He should just get over it and grow up."

I wasn't quite so sure, but I didn't want to think about it. It was much easier to go to Mass every morning and pray to God for Derek to seek forgiveness. He'd see that I wasn't a bad mother at all.

The moment when I died was the first time I blinked to see Derek one last time.

Sitting with a few other people around a long table in an Indian restaurant, Derek was holding a bald man's hand and laughing with him. I was stunned to see that he was with a *man*. Everyone at their table was quiet while a hearing woman shared a funny story about her father and his dog. She spoke and signed.

It was clear that some of the people at the table didn't sign, and some didn't speak. I was astonished by how civilized their conversation was. There were no interruptions. Ever.

Everyone listened.

That was a revelation.

Watching them, I envisioned a new kind of peace that I never knew could exist. The kind of peace that Jim and I never gave him. The kind of law and order we could've maintained at mealtimes, demanding that each person be heard with no interruptions.

I was surprised to learn that Derek was gay, but not quite so. He'd never spoken a word about who he was dating. I never asked.

Because I *knew*. Every mother knows.

But I didn't want to know.

Yet there it was: Derek was smiling radiantly. I had never seen such light emanating from any of my kids. His aura, lilting in soft rainbow hues, was quite warm and magnificent and powerful.

So much light! Who knew?

How could anyone have overlooked that about him?

And his boyfriend had a similar aura. Their auras throbbed together.

And I'd thought Derek dabbled in only resentment and darkness.

Watching my son, I knew what was coming next. His sister Carla had been trying to text him with the news that I'd died.

I'd been with her when I died in that awful hospital room. I hated the sound of my own heaves while trying to breathe.

In that disconnect between soul and body, the weight of cancer in my body was suddenly air.

I was flabbergasted by how freely I could move. I could slip through anything. Anyone alive I wanted to see, I was there in a blink.

That was how I blinked and found Derek. He looked older and a bit heavier than I recalled. It was still a shock to think of him as middle-aged, but he was. I had no idea what he'd done in the last five years before I died. I only hoped that he had been happy the whole time.

I blinked back to Carla, still trying to text. She was swearing to herself for not being able to reach Derek. I suddenly realized that he had to have blocked all of us from texting him.

Then I remembered that my youngest daughter Nancy would have his voice relay number.

I blinked back to Nancy. She had been sobbing. I whispered into her ear. "Try his voice relay number."

I blinked back to Carla just as her phone rang. It was Nancy. "Have you gotten ahold of Derek yet?"

"No! I think he's blocked me, too," Carla said.

"Okay. Let me try his voice relay number. Be right back."

I blinked back to Derek at the restaurant.

The man had just kissed Derek lovingly on the lips. He had a nice smile. I got the sense that these two were engaged to be married. I looked closely at the man. Was he good enough for my son? He looked to be about the same age as Derek.

Then Derek signed, *Marry where?*

I was startled by the fact that I could understand his signing perfectly. How was that possible? Did it mean that I had become all-knowing, like God?

Then Derek pulled his phone from his shirt pocket and set it against his wineglass. *Hi who call?*

I rushed to look at his screen. A woman in a black blouse was translating Nancy's voice into ASL. "Hi, Derek. This is Nancy. I just want you to know that Mom died a few minutes ago."

W-h-a-t? the interpreter voiced him.

"She had cancer in the bowels."

He paused. *W-o-w.*

"Yeah. Look, we're talking about having a funeral for her on Friday, so if you could come up by then, that'd be awesome. It'd be so good to see you."

Oh. Let-me think-about-it. Call-you b-a-c-k later will.

"Okay. We're still family. Remember that. Mom always wanted you to know that."

Rage flickered across his face as he slid the screen shut. *Family?* he signed to himself. *Hypocrites! W-t-f.*

His aura suddenly dampened into the graying and reddening colors of grief and anger. He looked ready to glow outward in the crimson of blood.

Who that? his boyfriend signed.

Derek signed and spoke at the same time. "My mother just passed away. Bowel cancer."

His friends signed awkwardly, *Wow so-sorry!*

His boyfriend slid around the table to sit next to him on the bench. He pulled Derek into his arms as my son sobbed.

Of course, I didn't want Derek to suffer, but it was satisfying to see that I was still a part of him, that he did have some feelings for me. I had long wondered if he still loved me.

It was all the proof I had needed.

The moment I died was the first time I began to grasp the full damage of what I'd done. Having no one alive on Earth to hear my lamentations was a new kind of hell.

I was that awful hearing mother who had thought learning ASL would be a waste of time.

I never asked him what *he* needed to be happy. How could I have been so selfish?

He didn't show up at my funeral. That really stung.

He's even changed his last name to his husband's.

He has thoroughly scrubbed his memory of me from his bones.

I am nothing. Not even a small puff of wind.

I have no voice left at the bountiful table of his life.

Here Lies the Body of a Deaf Boy

Here lies the body of a deaf boy
covered with a linen sheet of white,
centered perfectly atop the oval table
aligned under a vast half-moon lamp
in the kitchen. He is sweating
under the hot glare, the babbling
among the people encircling the table.
He knows just what they want
from having observed him. Their eyes
keep demanding in so many words.
He really is too much of a hassle.
Those ears are a real problem.
They love him, as siblings should,
but really, who wants to repeat anything?
Secondhanded jokes are no fun.
Such a party pooper! They want him
to suture back into the blankness
of the sheet clothing the table,
seating the plates, glasses, and silverware.
He needs to disappear just enough
into their gluttony of food and laughter
so none of them has to feel guilty
when they do not hear him laugh like they do.
Everything is silent, sterile, safe.
What it cannot lipread will hurt no one.

Decades Later in That Kitchen

The chain holding the half-moon lamp is cobwebbed,
graying the once-familiar landscape of the kitchen table
below where my siblings, white-haired, still cackle
over the jokes they think they've heard. It's clear
they're learning to play the game I once played.
The outline of my missing plate is a dust-free circle,
the absence of ghost at my spot on the bench.
It's been decades since I've returned to this house,
the very battlefield where I thought I'd died
over and over again in my rebirth of listening.
I never thought I'd see my siblings straining to hear,
but there they are, trying not to remember
how I'd survived this world with my hearing aids.
They'd never realized until then what an art
lipreading is, a stumbling passageway, a maze
filled with many wrong turns, a misunderstanding
at first trivial suddenly explosive: how they don't dare
don't mention how loud they need their TVs to be
or how grateful they are for the captions that appear
or how much they prefer to text than to talk on the phone.
They are too terrified to ask for their first audiogram.
I've become a dirty secret, a greasy reminder.
The more they babble, the more they try to talk over
each other, insisting that each other listen:
I am startled with a biblical revelation,
a flash of supernova radiating inside my eyes.
Could my deafness have enabled me to hear the world
far better than those with perfect ears
who haven't mastered the art of listening?
I decibel their cake slices with the syrup of frustration
having simmered with the sugar of misunderstanding.
They don't even notice it's *me* who's serving them.
They're that busy with pretending they have full hearing.
May their future hearing aids amplify the memory
of the deaf brother they've banished with neglect.

Deaf People Gather Kitchen For-For |
Why Deaf People Congregate in the Kitchen

[*in ASL gloss and English*]

kitchen lights bright always
not table over only no-no
everywhere also
stories share-share trade-trade same-same c-o-u-p-o-n-s
funny joke interrupt add
laugh-laugh-around
hands-sign-sign
shine warm-warm
remember-remember long-ago
time fight-fight hearing
time look-forward better world
{in-here-kitchen} chat-chat equal eat-eat thumbs-up
say-good-bye-around prolong-prolong {hands-over-heart}

*

The lights are always the brightest
not only over and beyond the table
where stories are traded like coupons
but also burnished with interjections
and chortles of laughter
until their hands are polished
with the patina of a time long gone
and the promise of a better time to come:
no better meal,
no sweeter long goodbye.

Washing the Dishes or What to Do While People are Talking

Dinner parties are, for me, a mixed bag. I love to cook and serve food to appreciative friends and family. I like the process of planning a menu, doing the shopping and the prep work and bringing food to the table. And of acourse, the best thing about a dinner party is having people come together for an evening of food and talk, but once I sit down, I experience what some deaf friends call Dinner Table Syndrome (DTS).

My experience of DTS as a late-deafened person with a small amount of hearing may be different from people who are congenitally or profoundly deaf. Depending on my interlocutor's pitch and vocal clarity, I can still make out some words and phrases, and thus have the illusion of participating in a conversation. But this is, indeed, an illusion since I can never successfully put together all the pieces of what's being said and have only a vague sense of its general subject. Topics change quickly, people interrupt or talk over each other. Just when I think I understand a reference and ask a question, the discussion has switched to something else. As someone said the other night, "Oh, we're not talking about that anymore."

The existential condition of DTS involves watching the crosstalk, laughter, and hilarity with bemused detachment. To be fair, my friends and family are quite solicitous, often pausing to ask if I'm "getting it," but then carrying on as before. When I become totally lost in the welter of words, I sometimes revert surreptitiously to reading email or Facebook posts. Finally, after an evening of struggling to understand what's happening, I end up washing the dishes—a therapeutic activity. My wonderful, sensitive friends and family do, after all, attempt to keep me in the loop, but after a while it's just too exhausting trying to keep up. Most irritating is when people turn away or cover their mouths or, assure me that "I'll tell you later what we're discussing." It's not that hearing people deliberately exclude me from the conversation but that in an oralist culture, no one thinks much about the embodied nature of language, the importance of lips, position, face and body language.

To make things easier, I use a captioning app on my iPhone called Ava which transcribes conversations on the screen. If others at the table have Ava on their phones, I can contact them via the app, and their voices appear in different colored fonts. Very helpful. But like all captioning services, Ava makes many errors and works most effectively in a one-on-one situation in a quiet space. In a crowded room with many people talking, the system breaks down. Restaurants, hotel lobbies, and airport waiting areas are impossible, and a dinner party is no exception. In such situations, Ava's screen is filled with wildly inventive errors and textual approximations of what is being said. As I have written elsewhere these errors often resemble avant garde poetry.[1] Here are a couple of samples taken at random from recent dinner table conversations:

I haven't the reason
the reason is a very popular topping in Taiwan
and a mini mini scholars have a being
devoted to their lives
to do the pizza and the Beast controversy
...
are you bye-bye hardback unkindly icy
by hardback that he finally got our bags
everything downtown La Jolla cool guy

As interesting as this language is, it's hardly satisfying as social exchange. Ava relies on Natural Language Processing (NLP) that uses algorithms to anticipate words in plausible sentences. It often recognizes (notice the paradox here: an "it" that can "recognize") an error of transduction and will correct "fuck" to "fruit," "ratatouille" to "rationale." When the system gives up, it usually translates the confusing phrase as "Hey, Siri," appealing perhaps to a higher digital power. People at the table often become fascinated by the errors the app makes and turn the conversation to Ava and its idiosyncrasies. I find this conversation especially weird, a bit like the one in which a salesperson addresses the caregiver rather than the person in the wheelchair.

This conversation between hearing people and app illustrates what I call "distributed voicing" to refer to the multiple ways voice is mediated, transcribed, transformed, and shredded. It also refers to the many ways that we now experience vocalization, whether through A.I. transcription systems, algorithms that transcribe words into text, machines that turn

---

1 *Distressing Language: Disability and the Poetics of Error.* New York: New York University Press, 2022.

text into voice like the one used by Steven Hawking, closed and open captioning, and sign language. My inclusion of the latter under the heading of "voice" might offend some deaf people since it implies that voice is configured under an oral ideology. That is, I may be imposing an audist value on Deaf cultural expression. The ASL sign for "voice"—the "V" handshape tracing up across the Adam's apple—may allude to the vocal cords within, but it can be used equally for expressive speech whether signed or spoken. ASL does have signs specifically for oral speech: "talk," a "4" handshape perpendicular to the mouth with small, repeated movements of the fingers, or "oral speech," a bent V handshape, moving in a small circular motion in front of the mouth. A related sign, "hearing person," involves the index finger moving in small rotations over the mouth. When the latter sign is repeated at the forehead, it transforms oral into "think hearing," an ideology based on the prioritization of sound and speech. All of which tends to reinforce my point that "voice" is distributed across multiple users and forms of communication. Voice is not a unitary phenomenon, owned and operated by hearing people, but a multimodal aspect of communication in general.

One final note. The deaf poet David Wright devotes a portion of his memoir to exhaustion.[2] He refers to how tired one becomes in situations like the dinner table context I've described. Straining one's eyes to read lips for two hours, looking back and forth across the table to catch a phrase, trying to give the impression that one is in on the joke—these factors can give one a headache. The analogy would be that of an English speaker with a smattering French or German, trying to understand a conversation in a bar or restaurant in that language. Such cross-cultural encounters produce a kind of linguistic enervation seldom discussed in accounts of sensory difference.

The phrase "Tell You Later" expresses a condition of deaf temporality where the context of a conversation—and by extension a person's agency—is deferred until after dinner when it can no longer be remembered.

---

2 Wright's memoir is written by a non-signing deaf poet who lost his hearing at age seven. He does not identify as culturally (capital "D") Deaf but, rather, as someone who continues to live in a hearing world. He acknowledges that "the recently deafened and lifelong-deaf have usually little in common" (127). True enough, but I think he misses an opportunity to seek commonalities along cultural, linguistic, and political lines. David Wright, *Deafness: An Autobiography*. New York: HarperCollins, 1993.

That Question Again

I have been asked again that loaded question: "Can you lipread?"

My answer was simply "No." I always reply that way.

The problem is that public perception of lipreading is not the same as my perception. If I answered "Yes," I would have to buy into their perception which is skewed in their favor, causing me significant hardship.

If I answered "Yes," the other party would just start talking without any consideration of light, clarity, pronunciation, accent, gesture, speed, sentence structure, and so forth. Therefore to ask that question without any intent to adjust their communication leads the original question to mean something very different.

"Can you lipread?" actually means "Can you do all the work of communication because I won't/can't/don't know how to make an adjustment to my own communication?"

Communication is a two-way process. It can't be one-sided.

Therefore, my reply to that question will always be "No." That answer challenges their preconceived assumptions about my ability to communicate and they are not let off scot-free. They will need to engage in the conversation fully with my support.

If we really want to change public perception, we all need to answer that question the same way. Just say "No."

They might look at you in disbelief because you have just answered their question. How could someone understand the question and still answer "No"?

The fact they are thinking about this is a pretty good start.

Waiting on the Next Big Thing

This week, on social media, I saw a Deaf influencer do a promotion of the latest technological innovation—AI live caption glasses. Cautiously optimistic, I clicked on the post, hoping that *this* would finally be the technology that would allow me to be a full-fledged member of my extended family of origin, all hearing, no signing. I clicked further and further into the post and saw how much the glasses cost, how much the monthly subscription cost. I closed the post, feeling once again the false seduction of technology and science. It's always out there, it's always coming soon, it's always shiny, and it's always way too expensive.

It's the next big thing that never arrives.

It's a broken promise between deaf people and their hearing families.

Yet it might be tempting for parents of young deaf children in the 21st century to say, surely, by now, deafness is a thing of the past, right? The utopian science fiction future is here or coming soon, so soon. We have, on the horizon, genetic engineering, along with a mechanism to deliver at least one genetic therapy for OTOF-gene-mediated hearing loss.[1] We've had cochlear implants for decades.[2] We've had hearing aids of different kinds for centuries.[3] The upwards trajectory of the development of technology and science has been so steep that hearing parents—past and present—might be tempted to think that we're already here in a future in which treatments and corrections and technologies should be at hand.

But the science of research into the genetic causes of deafness is still developing. While more than 90% of us are born to hearing parents, approximately 80% of prelingual hearing loss and 50% of

1   Alvin Powell, "Experimental Gene Therapy Enables Hearing in Five Children Born Deaf," News and Research, Harvard Medical School, 25 Jan. 2024, accessed 26 Aug. 2024. https://hms.harvard.edu/news/experimental-gene-therapy-enables-hearing-five-children-born-deaf

2   M Hainarosie, V Zainea, and R Hainarosie, "The Evolution of Cochlear Implant Technology and Its Clinical Relevance," PubMed Central (PMC), 2014, https://www.ncbi.nlm.nih.gov/pmc/articles/PMC4391344/

3   Hearing Health Foundation, "Hearing Aid History: Ear Trumpets, European Royalty, &Amp; Earbuds — Hearing Health Foundation," March 4, 2021, https://hearinghealthfoundation.org/blogs/hearing-aid-history-ear-trumpets-european-royalty-earbuds

all cases of hearing loss is currently thought to be caused by genetics or a combination of factors in addition to genetics.[4] The remaining percentage of deafness is thought to be caused by illness, trauma, and unknown factors.[5] Those of us who have no known history of hearing loss in the family are out there, being our deaf selves. We're a mystery to science. So, in addition to the proliferation of causes of deafness, gene "therapy" is likely not to be a pragmatic solution for most of us, despite what hearing parents may wish.

Other "options" are not always practical, either.

Then insurance doesn't always cover cochlear implantation, and when it does, the out-of-pocket cost may be cripplingly expensive.[6] After surgery, there's the need for follow-up therapies of different kinds, speech therapy, consonants and vowels and learning to discriminate sounds in the electronic waves surging through the cochlea hardware.[7] Additionally, there are multiple hidden costs that put cochlear implants out of reach for many families: the cost of transportation, the lack of flexibility in employment to schedule appointments, the variable cost of insurance co-pays, and so on. Even after all that, CIs are not guaranteed to work the way that hearing parents might expect: an implant is not a transplant. Dr. Wyatt Hall has researched the topic and concluded that "[s]igned languages are more effective at preventing language deprivation than cochlear implants are at remediating auditory deprivation."[8] There's much we already know about how science and technology is not an end-

4   "Quick Statistics About Hearing, Balance, & Dizziness," NIDCD, March 4, 2024, https://www.nidcd.nih.gov/health/statistics/quick-statistics-hearing, A Eliot Shearer et al., "Genetic Hearing Loss Overview," GeneReviews® - NCBI Bookshelf, September 28, 2023, https://www.ncbi.nlm.nih.gov/books/NBK1434/, Allen Young and Matthew Ng, "Genetic Hearing Loss," StatPearls - NCBI Bookshelf, April 17, 2023, https://www.ncbi.nlm.nih.gov/books/NBK580517/
5   Young and Ng, "Genetic Hearing Loss."
6   Stephanie Watson, "How Much Do Cochlear Implants Cost in 2024?," Forbes Health, March 6, 2024, https://www.forbes.com/health/hearing-aids/cochlear-implants-cost/
7   Cleveland Clinic Medical Professional, "Cochlear Implants," Cleveland Clinic, June 25, 2024, https://my.clevelandclinic.org/health/treatments/4806-cochlear-implants
8   Wyatte Hall, "Dry Hot Dog: Moving Beyond Auditory Deprivation," California EHDI Stakeholders Symposium, 11 Jan. 2020, CAD Collaborative & Educational Symposium Program Book, accessed 26 Aug. 2024, pp. 52-64, https://issuu.com/cad1906/docs/cadprogrambook-jan112020v2

all, be-all. With hearing aids, it's nearly the same set of issues, with the additional factors of discomfort and stigma related to hearing aids.[9]

Then there are the schools. Historically, it's been a struggle to fully fund, design, test, and implement accommodations for deaf and hard of hearing students due to a variety of factors. More recently, the school voucher movement threatens not to serve deaf and hard of hearing children.[10] Even if deaf and hard of hearing children and teens do pretty well in the classroom, there's always going to be something that they need support with, even if they tell you they are *fine, it's all fine, Mom.* Even if they "pass" for hearing or close enough some of the time. It's the other people you have to worry about, the teachers who mumble or talk to the board or get mad when your child can't help not hearing. And then anecdotal evidence from deaf and hard of hearing students suggests that they don't always receive appropriate IEP accommodations unless they are performing below grade level on school performance measures.[11] Generally, though, studies show that even well into the 21st century, deaf and hard of hearing children struggle to be on par with their hearing compatriots in relation to language, literacy, and numeracy.[12]

That science fiction future of *hearingness* is not here. It's always going to be out there, somewhere, always coming soon. But deaf utopia is already here. Hearing parents might know something about Nyle DiMarco, the winner of *America's Top Model, Season 22.* DiMarco went on to write a memoir with Robert Siebert, Deaf Utopia. DiMarco describes a specific lived experience, his own life within a multi-generational Deaf family. His Deaf utopia involves attendance at Deaf schools and 24/7 use of a fully accessible language, American Sign Language (ASL). One

9   Abby McCormack and Heather Fortnum, "Why do People Fitted with Hearing Aids Not Wear Them?" International Journal of Audiology 52, no. 5 (2013), 360-8, doi:10.3109/14992027.2013.769066

10 S. W. Cawthon, "Science and Evidence of Success: Two Emerging Issues in Assessment Accommodations for Students Who Are Deaf or Hard of Hearing," The Journal of Deaf Studies and Deaf Education 15, no. 2 (February 10, 2010): 185-203, https://doi.org/10.1093/deafed/enq002

11 Pamela Decker-Wright, personal communication, 30 Aug. 2024.

12 Shirin D Antia et al., "Language and Reading Progress of Young Deaf and Hard-of-Hearing Children," The Journal of Deaf Studies and Deaf Education 25, no. 3 (February 13, 2020): 334-50, https://doi.org/10.1093/deafed/enz050, L Gottardis, T Nunes, and I Lunt, "A Synthesis of Research on Deaf and Hearing Children's Mathematical Achievement," Deafness & Education International 13, no. 3 (September 1, 2011): 131-50, https://doi.org/10.1179/1557069x11y.0000000006

or more of these lived experiences is the utopia that a quarter-million to a half-a-million Deaf Americans experience.[13]

Those of us who were mainstreamed, who have CIs, hearing aids, and "learning to listen and speak" oral backgrounds, don't easily recognize ourselves in the Deaf world DiMarco writes about. The world we lived in was the spoken language world, a world we walked into on pathways painstakingly built from glimpses and fragments.

We have all experienced that sinking feeling at the dinner table or in the living room or at school when we, once again, don't know why everyone is laughing. Or we laugh too late or at the wrong thing. We know what it's like to have a family member or teacher say, "aw, that's so cute," when we mispronounce a word we read in a book or saw online. We feel jealous of the easy humor and jokes and teasing of DiMarco's world, the way that he had a close relationship and friendship with even his grandparents. Imagine!

But, driven by a desperate desire to understand, to belong, to know what's going on, those of us who entered the signing community later showed up at Deaf events, our hearts pounding. We borrowed sign language books from the library and downloaded sign language apps and practiced. We showed up.

It was hard sometimes. For those of us who were, at one time, "new signers," it never feels good to be the dunce in the room, the one that everyone has to slow down for. This is a lifelong experience no matter which language, at whatever age. It is awkward, and it is emotionally draining. But we kept showing up and showing up. Over time, we made friends and dated. We married Deaf people and adopted Deaf children or had children who signed, regardless of their hearing status.

We made it. It's not always the same neighborhood that DiMarco wrote about in his map of Deaf Utopia, but it's our home.

My own Deaf utopia is being able to relax, to look around and be able to understand my chosen family, all Deaf or signing. To make jokes or comment on what I know from what I've learned. To contribute. To be an equal member of the group at the dinner table.

---

13 Ross E. Mitchell, Travas A. Young, Bellamie Bachleda, "How Many People Use ASL in the United States?" Gallaudet Research Institute, Washington, D.C. Gallaudet University, 21 Feb. 2005, accessed 31 Aug. 2024, https://gallaudet.edu/wp-content/uploads/gcloud/gal-media/Documents/Research-Support-and-International-Affairs/ASL_Users.pdf

I'm fortunate to also be able to work in a bilingual setting where everyone knows sign language. It's not perfect. I'm not perfect. People are people, good, bad, boring, nice, mean, the same old stuff of being human. But I'm living in my utopia, my home, my work, my love, my life. I'm happy, at home, in a way that I could not have been if I was still stuck, still looking for the next big thing that would save me.

The last few times that I've visited my hearing family members, I tried out the new speech-to-text apps. I set out my phone on the dinner table, and watched the screen spit out words. Sometimes, full sentences, but then it dropped. Sometimes every third word, and then, in between, the other words would be gibberish. There's a reason why we call auto-generated captioning "craptions." Even AI can't hear well sometimes. Dinner Table Syndrome risks becoming a Dinner Table Life.

My own first foray into Deaf utopia began when I was in graduate school, struggling with falling further and further behind in just about everything. I've written about this experience elsewhere, so to sum up: a friend of my faculty advisor invited me to visit Gallaudet University. There, I met several Deaf adults, people who are now my friends and colleagues. It was a hard, long process to become fluent in ASL and to unlearn the hypervigilance and anxiety of *a dinner table life*, but I'm there now.

Recently, I told that friend, the same one who had invited me to visit DC all those years ago, that I could easily have had a so-so life, a *meh* life, a frustrating and inaccessible life. I was already on that pathway, that timeline. But because I felt desperate to make a change to my Dinner Table Life, I stepped out of that room, left that house, found my own neighborhood, my own home.

Now, I have a life that makes me feel lucky. Blessed, even.

Don't get me wrong. I love my hearing family of origin. I know they love me. No question. But it's hard to visit them and wish that I had truly effective live caption AI glasses. To feel once again, that sinking feeling of oh no, once again, I'm going to sit here for hours and hours, catching stray words here and there. I'm always happy to visit them because I love them. But I'm always quiet. It makes me wonder if they really know who I really am. And if I really know who they are.

It's a horrible feeling, to feel that way about people you love.

And not long ago, I visited a dear friend who is hard of hearing and who had married a hearing man who was excited to show off the signs he'd learned for her. A mutual friend, also deaf, joined me on this trip, and we sat together at their dinner table. He asked us what it's like to be deaf in a hearing world. The more my friends and I shared our stories with him, the more I could see him closing himself off, realizing that the story he'd been telling himself about us was not our experience. That the heart of our stories all had to do with *sharing*.

Not him *doing*. Doing a few signs for his new wife, a woman he looked at with his full heart in his eyes. Not him shaping his hands in a few slow signs, awkward, well-intended, the shapes becoming a shorthand for a whole world of meaning. Not him making sure that the light was on his face when he talked. Not him remembering to wait until his wife had put on her hearing aid. He did all of this diligently and with love. But he did this expecting her to always join him in his spoken, overheard life. No one can blame him for that. That's what a world of AI live caption glasses means.

What he didn't realize was that we were doing everything in our power to make it easy for *him*. We looked at his lips, shaping together what he meant, what he said, sharing with each other what we guessed he said. He didn't realize that real, full, free-flowing communication is shared. Sharing the conversation. Sharing the power. Sharing the responsibility. Sharing on equal footing.

And anyone who reads this collection already knows or knows by now the protoypical image of the dinner table syndrome: a young child sitting with their chin in their hands at a table filled with different dishes. It's usually a public holiday, Thanksgiving or Christmas. The meaning is clear. This child is being left out of the bounty, the family jokes, the snide comments, the inarticulate yammering of everyday talk, the ways that conversation moves over and around one's ears.

"But we're not really saying anything," they say when we ask. And as anyone who reads actual transcribed conversations knows, hearing-people-talk is filled with ums, hmms, yeahs, whatevers, and other stitched together pieces of a spoken life.

"What we're saying is nothing," they say, but if you pay attention the way we pay attention, you see the smiles, the nods, the laughs, the grimaces, the conspiratorial winks. You see the way that two people are bonding, the way two people are annoyed with each other. You see the fond smirks and the open-mouthed laughs, heads thrown back in delight. That's real, and that's what you share with each other.

For us, every day, every moment, becomes an unfunny, stressful, Mad Libs game. Constantly figuring out the context, predicting, praying for sudden onset of psychic skills, new technology, anything that would fill in the gaps.

I'm always grateful for whichever person realizes that I'm not following and relays a bit to me. Sometimes that's my mother, sometimes my sisters, sometimes my cousin, and sometimes my aunt. Always the women, acting out of the love they hold for me. But I can see that they have stepped out of the flow of the words to bring them to me. I love them for that, but I know that they can't do that the whole time. The table is not sharing.

So all of us who are living a Dinner Table life, we know that our families love us. They don't want us to feel left out. But we also know that simply by choosing not to share on equal footing, that's a decision. So we check out. We nod our heads, say a lot of "oh yeah, "oh cool," so that you don't feel the need to drop out of your own conversation to interpret once again for us. We remove ourselves by looking at our phones or at a book or at the TV. And over time, we don't visit as often. Or we make our visits shorter and shorter.

That's the most damaging part of the Dinner Table Syndrome—the feeling that you're a burden. An afterthought. This happens even when we can speak or kind of hear with a hearing aid or a cochlear implant. Even when there are family members who fingerspell the occasional word. We do a lot of faking it to make it easier for you because we love you, and we don't want to burden you. We make noises when it seems appropriate.

And this happens even with the kids whose parents and teachers think, "Oh, she can hear me just fine." And maybe we are getting something, sometimes, when we're not tired, when the lighting is good, when everything aligns.

But if you are a hearing parent of a deaf child, teen, or adult, have you asked yourself, "Just how often is my deaf family member faking understanding to make it easier for me and everyone else?"

Or have you asked yourself, "What am I doing that is encouraging my deaf family member to think that they should fake it to fit in or make it easier for everyone else?"

"Do you hear that?" my grandmother had asked me each time her bird clock chirped the hour. "Or that?"

Well, no, I didn't, but what was I going to tell her? It made me feel smaller and smaller each time she asked me just what I didn't hear. What I was not.

"Pretend like you're singing in church," my mother had said. "Just move your mouth to the words. Lip sync." This was after she told me in kindergarten how badly I sing, something I hadn't known before then. I had wanted to sing for Show and Tell. I know now she was trying to protect me from being laughed at, and she was my early champion and advocate. But I had loved singing, and it's one of the key silencing moments I remember from my childhood. Recently, she said that I sing better than my late-in-life hard of hearing stepfather, who apparently sings so horribly it's funny. What do I do with that information? Laugh?

"Don't do anything I wouldn't do," my father had said when he dropped me off at college. But he never talked to me. What would he not do? Now, years later, when I visit, he shouts my name at me, and my stepmother mumbles. We sit there for hours, watching TV and not talking. What we said could have been an email.

I love my family. I know they love me.

But we are not really able to share. To really talk back and forth. To laugh and be silly at nothing.

It breaks my heart to write this essay.

When I bring my signing, Deaf spouse and Deaf child (now an adult) to family gatherings, I always interpret for them as best I can, even with all the gaps and "I-have-no-idea-what-they-said." There's a reason I keep trying with different speech-to-text apps. I try to share as much as I can. I want them to feel even a little bit connected with the people who made me who I am.

As I get older, I choose to spend less and less time with my family of origin. It's too hard to be constantly faking it to make it easy for them, to be constantly a little bit left out. Especially when I'm in my Deaf utopia— my home and work—I am equal.

The point is that the deaf child at the dinner table grows up. If you are a hearing parent of a deaf or hard of hearing child, do you want them to have a dinner table life?

Will you be able to share with them after they leave home? When they introduce you to their beloved new partners, people who may be signing and not speaking? Will you be ready to navigate what happens when your grandchildren understand that you chose not to sign? Or chose not to work as hard as you could to become fluent?

Or, another story is that the child at the table grows up and partners with a hearing person, a person like my friend's husband. He's well-intended, sweet, loving, a good man, but they are not sharing on an equal footing. Are you ok with your now-adult child always being second, always being a beat behind?

Meanwhile, we all love each other with broken hearts and wait for AI live caption glasses. The next big thing.

Or the one after that.

The Deaf Table: a short play

DRAMATIS PERSONÆ

PERSON ONE – Twenty- to thirtysomething person. Deaf.
PERSON TWO – Twenty- to thirtysomething person. Deaf.

Behind an apartment building, an empty alley filled with garbage. ONE enters. They look around and sigh. They take out a vape and take a deep puff. As they slowly exhale, they look up thoughtfully at a window. Another draw. Another slow exhale. Finally, One sets about making a ramshackle seat from the surrounding garbage. It takes them a while. Finally, they sit and take yet another long draw.

TWO enters. For a moment, they stare at each other, unmoving. Then, exhaling, One gestures for Two to join them. Two nods gratefully and, as One watches, Two proceeds to build themselves a seat as well from the garbage. They sit in silence for a moment, connecting without speaking. Two makes to say something, but One interrupts, indicating that they are deaf. From here on, they sign in American Sign Language (ASL).

TWO   You're deaf?

ONE   Yeah. Are you?

TWO   Yep.

ONE   No shit?

TWO   No shit.

ONE   That's funny.

TWO   Hearing family?

ONE   Yeah.

TWO   Me too.

ONE   I'm sorry.

TWO   Me too.

ONE   Eighth floor.

TWO   Fifth.

ONE   Eleven people.

TWO   Seventeen.

ONE   Ugh.

TWO   Yeah.

ONE   All hearing?

TWO   All hearing.

ONE   Same.

        One offers Two their vape.

ONE   It's cranberry flavored. For the holiday.

TWO   Were they out of turkey?

ONE   I'm a vegetarian.

TWO   Ah.

With a grateful nod, Two takes the vape and draws long and deep.

ONE   That was a joke.

TWO   I know.

ONE   You didn't laugh.

TWO   It wasn't that funny.

ONE   Ouch. (Then, indicating the vape) Good?

TWO   Good enough. Thank you.

One nods. Two hands it back. Beat.

ONE   So where are you from?

TWO   New York City.

ONE   Busy.

TWO   Yeah. You?

ONE   Chicago.

TWO   Windy.

ONE   Yeah.

TWO   So what do you do? For work, I mean.

ONE   Publishing. I'm an editor.

TWO   Oh, nice. I'm reading this book now. Started it on the plane here, so I'm only about a third through so far. Saw it at the airport and thought it looked good, so I bought it.

ONE   What's it about?

TWO   This woman, she ... uh ... she goes on this long road trip with her dog and, uh ... they're at the Grand Canyon now and, um, the dog, he almost falls in, but this random guy shows up out of nowhere and saves the dog and now he's this big hero and ... um ... I think they're gunna fall in love. It's pretty obvious. You can see it coming a mile away.

ONE   *A Doggone Good Trip.*

TWO   Yes! Have you read it?

ONE   No, but we published it. My company, I mean.

TWO   Oh, that's funny.

ONE   Yeah. Small world.

TWO   Yeah.

        Beat.

ONE   What about you?

TWO   Hmm?

ONE   What do you do?

TWO   Oh. Right. I, um ... I work in advertising.

ONE   Cool.

TWO   Have you seen the new holiday campaign for Pepsi? With the penguins?

ONE   I love it. It's so cute.

TWO   My team created that.

ONE   Did you really?

TWO   Yeah. The cap that falls off and then ...

ONE   That's the best part!

TWO   Thank you. That was my idea.

ONE   Are you serious?

TWO   Yeah.

ONE   That's amazing.

TWO   Thank you.

ONE   Wow.

TWO   I was in the shower one day and it just came to me.

ONE   I get my best ideas in the shower too.

TWO   Who doesn't. That's why we have showers at the office. Whenever we hit a wall, we just jump in and lather up. Together.

ONE   Are you serious?

TWO   Yeah.

ONE   Really?

TWO   No!

ONE   Oh, okay! For a second, I was like ...

TWO   You thought I was serious!

ONE   No! I mean, well …

TWO   You did!

ONE   Maybe, but …

TWO   It's okay. I'm just having some fun with you. Anyway, it's become this big thing. The big joke around the office.

ONE   That's funny.

TWO   Yeah.

ONE   It really is.

TWO   I know.

ONE   So …

TWO   Speaking of funny …

ONE   Yeah?

TWO   It's funny how normal this feels.

ONE   Get out!

TWO   What?

ONE   I was just thinking that too. Seriously!

TWO   That's funny.

ONE   Yeah.

TWO   It feels …

ONE   Good.

TWO   Yeah.

       Beat.

ONE   If I can be honest, this is the first time I've had a conversation at Thanksgiving that went beyond, "You good?" and "Yeah."

       Above, the "You good?" and "Yeah." are both done via simple gestural conversation, such as a thumbs-up. It is very basic and superficial.

TWO   Me too.

       Beat.

ONE   This is the Deaf Table.

TWO   What?

ONE   Out here. With the garbage.

TWO   What do you mean?

ONE   Up there, my family's got two tables, one for the adults and one for the kids. They usually put me with the kids because I can't keep up / with the adults …

TWO   / Yeah, same here.

ONE   … but the kids aren't much better.

TWO   No, they're not.

ONE   But this table is the Deaf Table. Our table. For people like you and me. Where we can have a full, complex, adult conversation in our own language.

TWO   You know what else is kinda funny?

ONE   What?

TWO   The conversation we're having. I think most people, like hearing people, would say it was boring or nothing special ...

ONE   Yeah, because it's what they get to do all the time ...

TWO   Exactly!

ONE   But for people like you and me ...

TWO   We never get to do it.

ONE   Especially during the holidays.

TWO   Right. So this is nice.

ONE   Very nice.

TWO   Deaf people can actually do small talk, who knew?

ONE   Not our families, that's for sure.

TWO   I doubt if they even know that I worked on that penguin ad.

ONE   I bet most of them couldn't name any of the books I've worked on.

TWO   That's really sad.

ONE   I know.

> *Beat.*

TWO   It's starting to get dark.

ONE   Yeah.

TWO   Oh, by the way, did you hear about the tree lighting in town?

ONE   No. What happened?

TWO   Well, apparently, the person on the town board, or ... whatever, whoever's responsible for booking the company to string the lights on the tree just forgot to call them this year.

ONE   Oh, no.

TWO   Yeah, and I guess nobody followed up on it and it was this big oversight. And nobody realized until everyone was already at park for the annual tree lighting like two weeks ago, or maybe three, and, by then, it was too late. They're like, "We have no lights!" And / it's almost ...

ONE   / Wait a minute.

TWO   What?

ONE   I think that's what my family was talking about upstairs. I was trying to figure out what they were all ... but, yeah. Anyway, that's why I came down here. But I did catch one thing like ... there was a countdown or something?

TWO   Yeah! Exactly. So it's almost eight o'clock and everyone's got their scarves and hot chocolate and the crowd starts counting down —3, 2, 1—and the board or ... whoever's in charge, they finally realize and they're like, "Oh, shit!" There's no button or switch or whatever it is. And everyone's like yay! ... and they're just standing there waiting and waiting and ... of course, nothing happens. So they all kind of just … disperse, you know? Go home. So anticlimactic. Merry Christmas!

ONE   Oh, my God. That's insane.

TWO   Right?

ONE   Who told you about it?

TWO   I saw it on the news last night at the hotel as I was falling asleep. They were doing an update on the story. They finally got the lights up and tried to get people to come back and do it again, but most people were like, eh. So only like five people showed up.

ONE   That's so sad.

TWO   I'm not surprised, though. It's never as good the second time around.

ONE   No.

TWO   All the excitement is gone.

ONE   Exactly.

       Beat.

TWO   It may sound crazy, but … I'm just thinking here and, um … this might already be the nicest holiday I've ever had.

ONE   That's not crazy. I get it.

TWO   If not the most memorable.

ONE   Right. And, if I can be honest, I think it's true for me too.

TWO   Said as we sit here in an alley surrounded by garbage.

ONE   It's not the ambiance. It's the company.

TWO   Let's do it again at Christmas? You'll be here?

ONE   I'll be here. And now I actually have something to look forward to.

TWO   I'll bring the food.

ONE   I'll bring the wine.

TWO   Perfect.

> *One offers Two the vape again. Two takes it and draws. One takes it back and also draws. Together, they exhale.*

ONE   Well, I better go back in.

TWO   Me too.

ONE   I'll see you at Christmas?

TWO   I'll see you at Christmas.

> *They start to exit.*

ONE   Oh, wait.

TWO   What?

ONE   I never got your name.

TWO   And I never got yours.

ONE   Should we?

TWO   I don't know. Might ruin the magic.

ONE   I have an idea! If you show up at Christmas, I'll tell you then.

TWO   Deal. (Offering their hand)

ONE   Deal. (Taking Two's hand and shaking it)

With a mutual smile, they finally exit.

At My Table Now

My mom can sign.

I'm lucky.

They found out I was deaf.
Grandpa grew up next door to a Deaf guy who became an engineer.
He knew how to fingerspell.
Grandpa said, "Go find Deaf people. Ask them what to do."
Mom did.
She became an interpreter.

I am lucky.

She says she wanted us to have a relationship.
That worked. We are close.
She signed the nursery rhymes. She signed songs.
My friends were jealous.
But she also jokes
she wanted to make sure I knew
when she cussed me out.
But she signs to me.

So I am lucky.

Mom's eyes would glaze over when
she heard something across the room.
She'd laugh, eyes blank.
I could see she had stopped paying attention to my signs.
She said I didn't need to sign,
"I understand you, so just speak!"
I'm still not sure she listened.

But I was lucky.

I didn't know the strangers walking around the house.
I only knew their faces. Names.
Sitting on the porch. Playing in the backyard.
Every Christmas. Easter. 4th of July. Decoration Day.
We were visiting kin. Large. Loud. Talkative.
And Mom never signed around them.
None of them signed at all.
None of them understood my speech.
So I always sat alone, reading. Books never failed me.

I'm lucky.

At Mom's dinner table, my kids learned they didn't need to sign.
Not in front of the TV. Not on family trips. Not at the store.
Not at amusement parks.
But my kids can sign. Very well. They look Deaf.
My hard of hearing ex-husband signed. And spoke. Very well.
My mother's husband refused to sign.
Not even ILY.
They all didn't sign, even when I asked.

Their 10 ears and 5 mouths > 1 person.
My 53 years and 4 months > 1 person.

My kids grew up.
They now sign with and around and for me.
All the time. No matter what.
My hearing grandbabies sign.

I am lucky.

Gathering

Mingle Deaf, hear-ies
Laughter ensues, tell later
Later comes, train gone

"I'll tell you later."

No. Tell me NOW.

A.J. Chilson is a published poet and an award-winning children's book author. He was born in Dallas, Texas in 1984, and now lives and works in Winnsboro, Texas. A.J. has overcome the after-effects of childhood traumatic brain injury (TBI) and subsequent hearing difficulties to make his dreams in life come true.

Michael Davidson is Distinguished Professor Emeritus at the University of California, San Diego. He has written extensively on poetry and poetics (*The San Francisco Renaissance, Ghostlier Demarcations, Guys Like Us, On the Outskirts of Form*) and more recently on disability issues: *Concerto for the Left Hand* (University of Michigan), *Invalid Modernism* (Oxford University Press), and *Distressing Language: Disability and the Poetics of Error* (New York University Press). He is the editor of *The Collected Poems of George Oppen* and has published eight books of poetry, the most recent being *Bleed Through: New and Selected Poems* (Coffee House).

Pamela Decker-Wright is a dedicated ASL activist who has spent most of her life in language-related fields. She explored many different paths—teaching ASL, English, literature, and interpreting, and working with Deaf refugees, while staying connected to the theater and creative writing worlds. Pamela's short stories and poems found homes in *Deaf Way II Anthology, American Deaf Poetry: An Anthology*, and *American Deaf Prose*. Currently, she teaches linguistics at Gallaudet, and works on a project revealing more of ASL's superpowers! When she's not juggling her language passions, Pamela enjoys tending to her 57 plants, and maybe, just maybe, they can sign back!

Donald A. Grushkin is a graduate of Gallaudet University and the University of Arizona, where he received his doctorate in Language, Reading, and Culture. He is a Professor of Deaf Studies at the California State University, Sacramento. He lives in the San Francisco Bay Area with his wife, two children and one dog. A DTS survivor, he's been there, done that and has the full collection of T-shirts.

Kristen Harmon, born deaf to hearing parents, is now a professor of English at Gallaudet University. She has published short stories and creative non-fiction and is also an editor of multiple collections of creative writing written by Deaf people. Additionally, she has published scholarly articles on a wide range of topics from Deaf literature to narrative methodologies to Deaf bilingualism in education.

Cristina Hartmann is a DeafBlind Brazilian American writer living in Pittsburgh with her longtime partner and a slobbery cat named Moo-Moo. She received an MFA from the Vermont College of Fine Arts in 2024, and her work explores relationships and identity through disability and immigrant experiences. Her fiction was shortlisted for the *Masters Review* Summer 2021 Short Story Award and has appeared in Stillhouse Press's anthology *In Between Spaces*, *descant, Monkeybicycle, The MacGuffin, Peatsmoke Journal*, and elsewhere. [cristinahartmann.com]

Christopher Jon Heuer is the editor of *Tripping the Tale Fantastic: Weird Fiction by Deaf and Hard of Hearing Writers*. He is also the author of *Bug: Deaf Identity and Internal Revolution, All Your Parts Intact: Poems*, and numerous other short stories, articles, and poems. He is a professor of English at Gallaudet University in Washington, D.C.

Jer Loudenback has been Deaf since birth and the only Deaf member in his hearing family. A Washington state native, he moved to Minnesota after retiring as an ASL instructor and teacher of the Deaf. He is actively involved in numerous Deaf organizations, which he enjoys immensely. He has performed ASL poems, but this is Jer's second published work. He has enjoyed this process so much!

Raymond Luczak (Editor) grew up as the only Deaf child in his hearing family of nine children; he was not allowed to sign until he was fourteen years old. He is the author and editor of over thirty books, including *Animals Out-There W-i-l-d: A Bestiary in English and ASL Gloss, Assembly Required: Notes from a Deaf Gay Life*, and *The Language of Home: Stories* (forthcoming). His recent anthologies include *Yooper Poetry: On Experiencing Michigan's Upper Peninsula* and *Oh Yeah: A Bear Poetry Anthology*. He lives in Minneapolis, Minnesota. [raymondluczak.com]

Dominic McGreal was born in County Mayo, Ireland, and attended the boarding school for Deaf boys in Cabra, Dublin. After leaving school, Dominic dedicated his time and efforts to organizations such as the Deaf Men's Shed, Irish Deaf Youth Association, Dublin Deaf Association, Deaf Heritage Centre, Deaf Village Ireland, and Greenbow Deaf LGBT Society of Ireland. He served on the council of the Irish Sign Language Recognition. Since 1994, he has worked as an actor, director, and playwright at the Dublin Theatre of the Deaf. In 2002 Dominic received a Fulbright scholarship to study theater for one year at Gallaudet University. His passion for history led him to contribute short historical stories for the "An Conneal" book series, centered around his hometown of Louisburgh. He is the author of *The Revolutionary Lover*, a novel.

André Pellerin (Cover Artist) was born and raised in Vermont where he went to Austine School for the Deaf and graduated in 1976. Then he graduated with a double major in Theater Arts and General Psychology from Gallaudet University in 1982. He worked as a Technical Assistant to the Theater Department for over twenty years before transferring to the Art Department where he ran the gallery and assisted the ceramics program for ten years. After retiring in 2014, he joined the Red Dirt Studio in Mount Rainier, Maryland, where he was a member ever since. He died from complications due to liver cancer in 2024.

Kris Ringman is a deaf queer artist and author of *Sail Skin: poems* and two Lambda Literary Finalist books—*I Stole You: Stories from the Fae* and *Makara: a novel*. They often sit at dinner tables dreaming up their next poem, painting, or novel. Otherwise, they divide their time between painting murals in Portsmouth, NH, hiking in the White Mountains, flying to a far-off corner of the world, or on Block Island. [krisringman.com | IG: @wanderingnorsefox]

Doris Says grew up in a big family on Long Island. She is a multi-talented artist with a background in mixed media. She loves to read poetry, especially by Robert Frost, Maya Angelou, Edgar Allan Poe, Dorothy Miles, Clayton Valli, and others. She continues to create artworks that integrate nature, people, and landscapes.

Tonya Marie Stremlau has published a variety of short stories, including "Local Deaf Woman Abandons Twin Infants" and "A Nice Romantic Dinner." She is a professor in the English Department at Gallaudet University. She teaches a variety of classes, including creative writing, literature, and freshman composition. She is also the editor of the Deaf Lives Series for Gallaudet University Press. Outside of work, she is Mom to grown CODA twins and is obsessed with cooking and rock climbing. She lives with her husband just outside of Washington, D.C.

John David Walker is an academic leading a British Sign Language (BSL) and Deaf culture pathway as well as the Head of Department for language studies at the University of Sussex. He's also a human geographer who writes little snippets of thought from time to time on Deaf cultural capital, and walks in hand with his husband, Marco, by the sea in Brighton, with its white cliffs and heather.

Jacob Waring enjoys orbiting the planets of weird fiction, creating tales with a splash of space, mystery, and horror. He is a Southern Connecticut State University Journalism alumnus who contributed to the student section of "The Heart of the Coronavirus Crisis," which was published in the eight daily Hearst Connecticut newspapers and Insider websites. Waring has also contributed to the anthology *Tripping the Tale Fantastic: Weird Fiction by Deaf and Hard of Hearing Writers*.

Steven Wilhelm currently works as a lead analyst for Thoughtworks, from whom he has eagerly banked his paychecks for the last 24 years. He grew up with a moderate hearing loss that wasn't "discovered" until he was five years old. From age eight, he wore those alien body aids and depended heavily on lips. Fast forward to high skool where he taught himself rudimentary Sign. He didn't really grok Sign until his mid-twenties. Steven got his bilateral cochlear implants in his mid-fifties. Half-hearing, half-deaf … He complains it's so confusing at times! Steven calls the Mojave Desert home.

Rachel Zemach, after thirteen years of teaching Deaf students in a hearing public school, wrote a memoir in order to describe her joyful but also shocking experiences there, and start a national dialogue about mainstream Deaf education. In *The Butterfly Cage*, readers meet individual students, watch raucous and often surprising class discussions, and see her personal journey as her identity undergoes dramatic shifts. She lives in North California with a husband who doesn't sign very well—which may be why he introduces her as his "hamburger" when signing—and a bossy cat named Puppy. [rachelzemach. com]

Garrett Zuercher (he/him) earned his MFA in playwriting from Hunter College and has seen his award-winning plays produced at such world-class venues as the Kennedy Center and The Shed. When not writing, he serves as the founding artistic director of Deaf Broadway and directs many of their stage productions at Lincoln Center. He is an actor and filmmaker as well; his cinematic creations continue to garner honors at film festivals around the world. Dedicated to bringing authentic Deaf voices to the mainstream, he is a staunch advocate for awareness and representation within the theater and film industries. [garrettzuercher.com]

www.ingramcontent.com/pod-product-compliance
Lightning Source LLC
Chambersburg PA
CBHW071018130325
23443CB00027B/251